Medical Library

Queen's University Belfast
Tel: 028 9063 2500
E-mail: med.issue@qub.ac.uk

For due dates and renewals:

QUB borrowers see 'MY ACCOUNT' at
http://library.qub.ac.uk/qcat
or go to the Library Home Page

HPSS borrowers see 'MY ACCOUNT' at
www.honni.qub.ac.uk/qcat

This book must be returned not later
than its due date but may be recalled
earlier if in demand

Fines are imposed on overdue books

The most common, most easily recognised and probably the most researched single condition causing learning disability is Down's syndrome. On the basis of extensive tests, interviews and questionnaires focusing on fundamental issues of development and upbringing, Dr Carr has followed the lives of a population-based cohort of people with Down's syndrome from birth to early adulthood. This volume details particularly the development of the study groups at the ages of 11 and 21 years with a longitudinal perspective reference to earlier years as appropriate. A wide range of factors are investigated, from abilities, behaviour, discipline and independence through to effects on the family and the provision of help from services. The collection of these unique data spanning the first 21 years of life enables Dr Carr to offer discussion and advice that will be of international relevance and an invaluable reference for all those concerned with the care, health and well-being of individuals with Down's syndrome and their families.

Down's syndrome

JANET CARR

Down's syndrome
Children growing up

*The author was formerly Regional Tutor in the Psychology of Disability,
St George's Hospital Medical School, London*

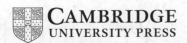

CAMBRIDGE
UNIVERSITY PRESS

Published by the Press Syndicate of the University of Cambridge
The Pitt Building, Trumpington Street, Cambridge CB2 1RP
40 West 20th Street, New York, NY 10011–4211, USA
10 Stamford Road, Oakleigh, Melbourne 3166, Australia

© Cambridge University Press 1995

First published 1995

Printed in Great Britain at the University Press, Cambridge

A catalogue record for this book is available from the British Library

Library of Congress cataloguing in publication data

Carr, Janet H.
Down's syndrome : children growing up /
Janet Carr.
    p. cm.
  Includes index.
  ISBN 0 521 46532 X (hbk.). – ISBN 0 521 46933 3 (pbk.)
  1. Down's syndrome – Patients – Longitudinal studies. I. Title.
RJ506.D68C36   1995
362. 1'96858842 – dc20   94–46986 CIP

ISBN 0 521 46532 X hardback
ISBN 0 521 46933 3 paperback

To all the young people, and their families, who have been my friends since 1963 and have taught me so much.

CONTENTS

Acknowledgements

The 11 year phase of this study was carried out while the author was on partial leave of absence from the Department of Psychology, Institute of Psychiatry, University of London; and the 21 year phase while the author was employed in the Departments of Psychology and Psychiatry of Mental Handicap, St George's Hospital Medical School, London, and was supported at this time by a grant from the University of London Central Research Funds Committee.

I am deeply grateful to Professor Joan Bicknell who insisted that the 21 year study must go ahead; to Dr Glyn Murphy who read the first draft of the manuscript and made many helpful comments; to Dr Sheila Hewitt who participated in the 11 year study, interviewing most of the families of the children with Down's syndrome, and also read and commented on the first draft of the manuscript. Finally I feel forever in the debt of the late Professor Jack Tizard who guided me through the earlier stages of the study, and who would I think have been pleased to see it continue.

Pg 1 → D.S.

Incidence, characteristics

etc.

GABITRIL
Tiagabine

ONE

Down's syndrome – implications of the diagnosis

D own's syndrome is the most common, the most easily recognised and probably the most researched single condition causing learning disability. It was first identified by John Langdon Down in 1866; almost certainly it had existed long before that, possibly as far back as the seventh century (Brothwell 1960), while some sixteenth and seventeenth century paintings have depicted infants with 'mongoloid features' (Cone 1968; Zellweger 1968). Zellweger, however, warned of the dangers of accepting this kind of pictorial evidence, pointing out that the infant shown in one such painting later went on to become an admiral of the British Fleet. Richards (1968) suggested that the condition may indeed have been rarer in the past because of smaller populations and higher rates of infant and maternal mortality, and the fact that in the mid-nineteenth century only 58% of women survived to the age of 35, which, as this is the high risk age for mothers of Down's syndrome babies, would have reduced the incidence at that time.

Down (1866) expounded his theory that many of the patients he saw, both in the Earlswood Asylum and as out-patients, could be identified as belonging to one or other of the ethnic groups: Caucasian, Ethiopian, Malayan, from the South Sea Islands and from the American continent. He drew particular attention to 'the great Mongolian family' and gave a detailed description of them:

> The face is flat and broad, and destitute of prominence. The cheeks are roundish, and extended laterally. The eyes are obliquely placed . . . [and] the palpebral fissure is very narrow. . . . The lips are large and thick . . . the tongue is long, thick and much roughened. The nose is small. . . .
> They are always congenital idiots, and never result from accidents after uterine life . . . [and they] very much repay judicious treatment. They have considerable powers of imitation, even bordering on being mimics. They are humorous, and a lively sense of the ridiculous often colours their mimicry. They are usually able to speak; the speech is thick and indistinct, but may be improved greatly by a well-directed scheme of tongue gymnastics. The coordinating faculty is abnormal, but not so defective that it cannot be greatly strengthened. By systematic training, considerable manipulative power may be obtained. . . . The improvement

which training effects in them is greatly in excess of what would be predicated if one did not know the characteristics of the type. The life expectancy, however, is far below the average.

Thus, Langdon Down not only gave a description of the people whose condition now bears his name but also drew attention to a facet of their makeup – their responsiveness to and the benefit they can derive from teaching and training – that was largely ignored for about a century.

Incidence, prevalence and life expectancy

Incidence (the number of babies born) is commonly given as 1/600 live births (Wishart 1988). This is an approximation, or average figure, and recorded incidence has varied from time to time. In the city of Salford, where incidence was particularly carefully monitored, it dropped from 1/565 in 1961–65 to 1/1075 in 1971–75, and then rose to 1/730 in 1976–80, showing a 'periodicity' that is seen also in other studies (Fryers 1984). As is well known, incidence varies with maternal age, rising from 1/1600 at age 20–24 to 1/100 at 40–44 and 1/46 over the age of 45 (Collman & Stoller 1962). Slightly different figures are given in other reports but all show the rise with maternal age (Hook 1976). The effect of paternal age is unclear: Zaremba (1985) quoted the opinion of Penrose (1933) that paternal age was of no significance, followed by that of Stene *et al.* (1981) that it had an effect that was independent of maternal age, later still by the opinions to the contrary of other workers (Hook & Cross 1982; Ferguson–Smith 1983), leading Zaremba finally to the endorsement of 'the rightness of the original conclusion of Penrose (1933)'.

In the 1970s there was a drop in maternal age for all mothers and this was mirrored by that for mothers of babies with Down's syndrome (Owens *et al.* 1983); after 1971 over 70% in Scotland were aged less than 35 (Murdoch 1982). More recently the trend has once more reversed, and figures have shown an increase in such births to women over the age of 35 (Holloway & Brock 1988), with the possibility that incidence might again rise.

The effect of prenatal diagnosis

Towards the end of the 1960s it became possible to screen pregnant women for a number of disabling conditions, including Down's syndrome. In 1973 it was proposed that complete prevention of Down's syndrome could be achieved by screening every pregnancy by amniocentesis and karyotyping of the foetal cells (Stein, Susser & Gutterman 1973). Such a programme has never been established but screening is commonly available to older women, that is women of 35 or over, and to women at special risk (i.e. with a relative with Down's syndrome). Even with this limited availability there was an expectation that the incidence of Down's syndrome would decline, independently of other influences such as a fall in the general birth rate. These expectations have not been met, and hitherto the effect of pre-natal diagnosis on incidence has been slight. The reasons for this include the following:

1. The age of mothers offered screening. Although the incidence of Down's syndrome is higher in older mothers, because they have a relatively small number of babies compared with those born to younger mothers the majority of babies with Down's syndrome – around 70% (Murdoch 1982; Steele 1993) – are born to younger mothers, who are not included in most screening programmes.

2. Low rates of take-up of screening. Rates vary considerably, but over a 10 year period (1976–86) take-up reported from a number of UK centres averaged only about 25%, although it tended to increase over the years (Steele 1993).

3. Some women who are eligible for screening refuse, on moral or religious grounds (Ferguson-Smith 1983) – or because they are unwilling to take the risk (estimated at about 1–2%, Stein *et al.* 1973; British Medical Journal 1977) of damage to or abortion of a potentially healthy foetus (Knight 1988).

It seems unlikely that the numbers of babies born with Down's syndrome will be much reduced in the near future, although all this may change with the development of new, more effective, more economical and safer methods of prenatal diagnosis: for example, the 'quadruple' test, which, used in con-junction with routine screening, is able to detect over 65% of affected preg-nancies, with only a 5% false positive rate (Wald & Watt 1994).

Prevalence, the number of people with Down's syndrome alive in the community at any one time, varies according to the age group under con-sideration and is always highest at the earliest ages, declining as some infants and young children, and smaller numbers of adolescents and adults, die. Early in this century, when mortality among children with Down's syndrome was high, by school age (7–14) they constituted only 0.34/1000 of the population of that age group. In 1929 the proportion had increased more than three-fold to 1.4/1000 (Goodman & Tizard 1962). In the Sal-ford studies, prevalence of 5–14 year olds rose steadily to a peak of 1.48/1000 in 1973 and declined thereafter, due probably to the fall in the birth rate (Fryers 1984, pp. 102–3). Since survival to one year is now of the order of 80–90% we may expect to find over 5000 teenagers with Down's syndrome alive in the year 2010, and figures from both this country and others indicate that 'throughout the next century the population prevalence of Down's syndrome will be higher than ever before' (Nicholson & Alberman 1992). Contrary to trends seen in the general population, males commonly outnumber females, rates quoted being between 1.07:1 and 1.27:1 for 0–4 year olds (Fryers 1984) and 1.28:1 and 1.36:1 for whole populations (Stratford & Steele 1985). This sex difference may be due to higher mortality in females, especially in infancy (Gibson 1978, p. 104).

The commonly held view of Down's syndrome as involving a short life-span was, until the last half century, quite accurate. In 1929, life expectancy (the average length of life of all those born with the condition, including those dying at birth or in infancy) was estimated as 9 years, and by 1947 had increased to 12 years (Penrose & Smith 1966). Few people with Down's syndrome lived to be mature adults: in 1947, of 138 cases known to five local authorities, only 6% were over age 34 and none over 45 (Penrose 1949). Since then, however, recent studies have shown a continuing rise in life expectancy, brought about largely through the increased survival of infants and young children. Sixty per cent of children born between 1940 and 1950, 80% born between 1950 and 1970 and 90% born between 1976 and 1985 reached at least their first birthday, while the figures for those reaching their fifth birthday were 42%, 71% and 79%, respectively (McGrother & Marshall 1990). It is now estimated that nearly half (44%) of those born between 1952 and 1981 will survive to age 60 and 13.6% to age 68 (Baird & Sadovnik 1988). These figures are well below those for the general population (86.4% of whom survive to age 60 and 76.4% to age 68) but it is likely that they are considerably higher than they were in the past. Over the last 50 years the lifespan of hospitalised people with Down's syndrome has increased by an average of 40 years (Jancar 1988) and people with Down's syndrome over the age of 60 are now 'not exceptional' (Dupont, Vaeth & Videbech 1986). Nearly two decades ago the oldest person with Down's syndrome who could be traced at that time was aged 65 (Carr 1975); a more recent claimant to that title is a woman of 75 (Demissie, Ayres & Briggs 1988), outdone in her turn by the oldest of 'at least three persons with DS [Down's syndrome], 74, 75 and 86 years of age respectively, presently alive and leading healthy lives with no apparent evidence of impairment or deterioration' (Dalton & Wisniewski 1990).

Characteristics

Cognitive

The physical characteristics of people with Down's syndrome are well known, and full descriptions of them may be found elsewhere (Penrose &

Smith 1966; Kirman 1975). (Mentally, the principal characteristic for the majority is learning disability.) In the early weeks of life average ability measures are somewhat below the norm for babies generally and then decline (Carr 1985). This decline in IQ does not indicate that, as they grow older, people with Down's syndrome become less competent: their mental age (MA) continues to increase, and they continue to learn and to develop skills. After the first few years (2–4) the rate of decline slows and the trend may even reverse in adulthood (Berry *et al.* 1984; Fenner, Hewitt & Torpy 1987; Carr 1988a). The reasons for the decline in IQ have been much debated. Early theories postulated a deterioration in cerebral function (R. Griffiths, personal communication, reported in Kirman 1969; Dicks-Mireaux 1972), others that it might be due to the increase in the emphasis on language in later tests (Bilovsky & Share 1965; Melyn & White 1973). In most studies, however, the most rapid decline takes place before 3 years (when tests are weighted with non-verbal items) and continues more slowly after that, when tests become more verbally loaded. Gibson (1978, pp. 30–34) suggests that several factors may contribute to the decline. Specific neuromotor and sensory disabilities may emerge only as the infant grows older; the Down's syndrome child appears to have greater difficulty in 'bridging the gap' between sensory-motor and cognitive performance than has the non-disabled child; the decline may be 'a result of progressive or central nervous or system arrest or is an expression of a growing deficiency of the sensory and expressive periphery' and Gibson warned against facile acceptance of the cerebral deterioration hypothesis. The reasons for the decline, then, are still not clear.

Of the different types of Down's syndrome, the most common is standard Trisomy 21 (G) the others being translocations involving chromosome groups D/G or G/G, which account for about 4% of the population with Down's syndrome. Mosaicism, in which not all the cells show the chromosomal abnormality, can occur in either case and is found in about 3–4% of the population with Down's syndrome (see Kirman 1975, pp. 128–133). Children with the mosaic form of the condition have been assessed as having mean scores that are higher than the means of those with standard Trisomy 21 (Kostrzewski 1974; Gibson 1978, p. 81). Fishler & Koch (1991) also noted this superiority and claim that it is maintained into late adolescence. This paper is confusing: the data presented in Table I and Figure 1 are, although this is not stated, based on different populations (K. Fishler, personal communication), and there are inaccuracies in several of the figures given. However, these anomalies do not affect the main argument of the paper. Regardless of the type of Down's syndrome, a wide range of abilities is demonstrated, of the order of 50–60 IQ points, in both children and adults (Carr 1988), showing that people with Down's syndrome differ one from another to an extent similar to that seen in the non-disabled population.

Females are consistently found to have higher average scores than do males, whether as children (Wallin 1944; Carr 1975; Clements, Bates & Hafer 1976; Connolly 1978; Carr & Hewett 1982; Cunningham 1987) or adults (Pototzky & Grigg 1942; Carr 1988a), apart from one study in which there was no difference between the sexes (Ramsay & Piper 1980). Various explanations have been put forward for the higher scores of females: that the presence of the XX sex chromosome 'may tend to reduce the severity of measured mental retardation within . . . Down's syndrome children' (Clements *et al.* 1976); that parents may interact differently with their Down's syndrome sons and daughters (Connolly 1978); that it may be due to the greater linguistic facility of females (Schnell 1984; Cunningham 1987); and that selective mortality may be responsible, with more vulnerable females dying earlier whereas similarly disabled males continued to survive. None of these explanations has proved entirely convincing and the reason for the superiority of females remains undecided. It should be noted, however, that it relates to average figures, and that amongst individuals the full span of ability is seen in members of both sexes.

Early intervention

One of the most hopeful developments in the last 25 years has been the application of early stimulation and training to infants and young children with Down's syndrome. Interventions have varied in the type of programmes, length of time they lasted, numbers of children and frequency of training sessions involved, and evaluation methods used. With one exception (Piper & Pless 1980), all report advantages to the children in the programmes. Clearly this is what those working in the field expect and hope for. However, there is still need for caution. Most of the published studies are methodologically less than satisfactory (Carr 1992b) and long-term studies showing the maintenance of initial advantage are lacking (Gibson & Harris 1988). Effective intervention has commonly been reported while the intervention was ongoing, and Cunningham (1987) documents the failure of such effects to survive the termination of the intervention. At present there is no published evidence to show the effects of early intervention programmes on the lives of the children when they become adults, although this may well be forthcoming in the future.

Personality

Much discussion has centred on whether the popular view of people with Down's syndrome as cheerful, friendly, imitative, affectionate and fond of music (Tredgold 1937) has any basis in fact. Some early work stresses their variability (Rollin 1946), while Blacketer-Simmonds (1953) counters the stereotype by finding them less docile and more mischievous than were other people with learning disabilities, and no difference between the groups in their responsiveness to music. Others have found some support for the stereotype, hospital residents with Down's syndrome being significantly more often positively rated by nurses (Silverstein 1964), and these findings were supported in other studies (Ellis & Beechley 1950; Domino, Goldschmid & Kaplan 1964; Domino 1965; Johnson & Abelson 1969). More recent work stresses the normality of the range of temperament in toddlers with Down's syndrome (Baron 1972) and the changes, predominantly positive, that occur between infancy and childhood (Gunn, Berry & Andrews 1981, 1983; Gunn & Berry 1985). The process was taken further with research on older children, aged 8–14, who were shown to be more predictable, more positive in mood, less active and persistent, and more distractible than non-disabled children (Gunn & Cuskelly 1991). When the children were divided into those above and below 11 years, the older group were similar to the younger but more predictable and persistent, failing to substantiate Gibson's suggestion that the pleasant child with Down's syndrome 'turns subsequently into a sullen adolescent'. Gibson (1978, p. 148) adds, however, 'but not always and maybe not even in the majority of instances'.

A recurring question has been how far the stereotype is self-fulfilling; how far the ratings of personality in people with Down's syndrome are influenced by the raters' awareness of the stereotype. Mothers of children with Down's syndrome, who might be regarded as likely to be realistic about the condition, provided broader descriptions than did mothers of non-disabled children but with a very similarly positive content (Rodgers 1987). Results from a study by Wishart & Johnston (1990) are in close agreement: in general, the more experience the study participants had of children with Down's syndrome the less they adhered to the stereotype. However, the highest (most stereotypical) ratings were given by mothers of their own children, and by special needs teachers. The authors suggest that this may be due to the predominantly positive nature of the stereotype, both these groups being likely to have a positive approach to children with Down's syndrome. In general, however, the notion that mothers who live with the daily reality of Down's syndrome would dismiss the stereotype has so far failed to gain much support.

Silverstein *et al.* (1985), in one of the few recent papers to include consideration of the personality of adults, and again finding support for the favourable stereotype, suggest that the effect may have been indirect. Carers who subscribe to the stereotype may have adapted their own behaviour in such a way that they brought out the best in the people with Down's syndrome with whom they interacted, a suggestion which, if substantiated, indicates directions for the training of all care staff – and, perhaps, many others besides.

Health

Physical health

People with Down's syndrome are often thought of as fragile and sickly, and indeed they are prone to some particular ailments. Most, however, are rated by those closest to them as being in good health, whether as children (Carr 1975), teenagers (Buckley & Sacks 1987) or adults (Shepperdson 1992), although medical problems, especially skin problems which affected about a quarter, were more frequent than in non-disabled people. Else-where, poorer health, compared with controls, has been reported (Turner *et al.* 1990), although this did not result in the children being off school unduly often. Problems with vision have been found in 49–71% (Buckley & Sacks 1987; Turner *et al.* 1990; Shepperdson 1992), with lower figures, below 30%, given in some adult surveys (Holmes 1988; Myers & Pueschel 1991). Estimates of hearing difficulties range from 8% to 26% (Buckley & Sacks 1987; Turner *et al.* 1990; Myers & Pueschel 1991; Shep-perdson 1992) but higher levels, of 38% in an institutionalised population (Jancar 1988) and 48% in those over the age of 50 (Hewitt, Carter & Jancar 1985), have been reported. It may be that the extent of these diffi-culties is being underestimated (Buckley & Sacks 1987; Cunningham & McArthur 1981), and certainly where hearing is assessed by means of proper tests, rather than through estimates made by carers, higher levels of difficulty tend to be discovered, i.e. 43% (Yeates 1992) and 69% (Nolan *et al.* 1980). About half of young adults are overweight, this being almost twice as common in women as in men, and the proportion who are over-weight increases to about two-thirds of those in their mid and late twenties (Holmes 1988; Shepperdson 1992) whereas even higher levels, of 81% overweight or obese, are reported for a group with a mean age of 44 (Prasher 1994).

Heart problems affect about half of all babies with Down's syndrome (Hallidie-Smith 1985) and in the past were responsible for many of the early deaths. Between 25–40% of older children and adults are affected (Rowe & Uchida 1961, citation from Gibson 1978; Myers & Pueschel 1991). Epilepsy is relatively unusual, affecting fewer than 15% (Corbett 1973; Holmes 1988; Shepperdson 1992). Thyroid deficiency is much more common in people with Down's syndrome than in non-disabled popu-lations, though the frequency with which it has been found has varied widely in different studies, from 0 to 66% (Prasher 1994). The incidence of cancer appears to be similar to that in the general population, apart from an increased risk of childhood leukaemia (Thase 1982b).

Overall most people with Down's syndrome enjoy reasonably good health, although heart, thyroid, skin and sensory problems may be troublesome.

Mental health

People with Down's syndrome are not immune to psychiatric illnesses, but compared to people with other forms of learning disabilities they are relatively mildly affected. In one study the proportion of people with Down's syndrome with any kind of mental illness was 22%, well below the 32–59% found in those with other forms of learning disability (Myers & Pueschel 1991), and they appear to be less vulnerable to many psychiatric illnesses – conduct disorders, neuroses, schizophrenia/paranoia (Collacott, Cooper & McGrother 1992), females being particularly lightly affected (Lund 1988). Depression, however, may be more common in people with Down's syndrome, seen in 11% compared with only 4% of those with other forms of learning disability, with a mean age of onset of 29 years (Collacott *et al.* 1992). Depression is especially important in people with Down's syndrome since it may either mask, or be misdiagnosed as, dementia (Warren, Holroyd & Folstein 1989). A number of cases have been successfully treated with ECT (electroconvulsive therapy), following failure to respond to medication (Lazarus, Jaffe & Dubin 1990). Mania has been thought to be incompatible with Down's syndrome (Sovner, Hurley & LaBrie, 1985) but some well-attested cases have been described (Cook & Leventhal 1987; Haeger 1990; Cooper & Collacott 1991). Folie à deux in a 29 year old man and his 77 year old mother was successfully treated (Meakin, Renvoize & Kent 1987), but obsessive-compulsive disorders were more resistant (O'Dwyer, Holmes & Collacott 1992). Anorexia has been reported (Cottrell & Crisp 1984; Szymanski & Biederman 1984), with in one case an account of successful treatment through the application of behavioural techniques (Holt, Bouras & Watson 1988). Self-injury is relatively rare in people with Down's syndrome (Myers & Pueschel, 1991; Carr, 1992b); in one of the few cases reported in the literature a rapid and dramatic response to a diet high in serotonin is described (Gedye 1990).

The effects of ageing and Alzheimer's disease

Signs of ageing occur early in people with Down's syndrome, and the connection between Alzheimer's disease and Down's syndrome, 'a sort of precipitated senility', was first noted by Fraser & Mitchell in 1876, followed later by the identification, in the brains of people with Down's syndrome, of the characteristic plaques of Alzheimer's disease (Struwe 1929). These neuropathological signs have been considered to be present in the brains of all people with Down's syndrome over the age of 40 (Thase 1982b), or even earlier (Heston 1977; Wisniewski, Wisniewski & Wen 1985). (An excellent review of the principal features of Alzheimer's disease and Down's syndrome is given by Oliver & Holland (1986).

While there is some debate as to the age at which it may appear, there is no doubt that Alzheimer's disease occurs earlier in people with Down's syndrome than in the general population. Much less clear cut are the findings on the appearance of the cognitive and behavioural changes that are usually associated with such neuropathology. The changes that are commonly seen in people with Down's syndrome have been summarised by Oliver & Holland (1986) as: behavioural (becoming 'unmanageable' or withdrawn), loss of self-care skills, deterioration in the use or understanding of language, apathy, and later complete helplessness. It is important to remember, however, that a number of other conditions, such as visual and hearing problems (Hewitt *et al.* 1985), depression (Warren *et al.* 1989) and hypothyroidism (Thase 1982a) can mimic dementia, and should always be considered if dementia is suspected, especially in a young person.

Research projects concerned with the assessment of these changes have involved tests of intelligence and memory, and the assessment of daily living skills.

Intelligence tests carried out on cross-sectional samples have shown lower scores in the majority of those over the age of 45 (Hewitt *et al.* 1985; Fenner *et al.* 1987). Using a variety of tests of orientation, object identification and visual memory, Thase and his colleagues showed that the scores of institutionalised people with Down's syndrome declined with increasing age, particularly on the memory tests, although the same effect was not seen in other IQ-matched hospital residents (Thase 1988). Longitudinal studies showed that memory function began to fail at an average age of 49 (Dalton & Crapper-McLachlan 1984), and deficits were apparent when not only the more usual auditory but also visual material was used (Marcell & Weeks 1988). Poorer performance with increasing age has also been found where practical and daily living skills are concerned, but there were few differences between people with Down's syndrome and those with other forms of learning disabilities, apart from poorer eating skills and mobility in the group with Down's syndrome, and that only for those over the age of 60 (Silverstein *et al.* 1986); while in a longitudinal follow-up the only difference seen was, again, that of greater decline in mobility in the Down's syndrome group over age 50 (Silverstein *et al.* 1988). Other research on changes in daily living skills has supported these findings, showing greater fall-off in the skills of those with Down's syndrome, but not until after age 50, and becoming more pronounced after age 60 (Zigman *et al.* 1989; Collacott 1992).

In summary, most research reveals little evidence of deterioration in IQ, memory or practical skills in the majority of people with Down's syndrome before the age of 50, or in some cases 60, well beyond the age at which the neuropathological signs of Alzheimer's disease are commonly found in this population. Moreover, fewer than 50%, even in the oldest age groups, show clear signs of dementia (Thase 1988). A variety of reasons have been put forward to account for these divergent findings: inadequate test procedures, the 'floor effect' (that is, the low scores in profoundly learning-disabled people might prevent any decline being observable; Oliver & Holland 1986), and whether there is a prolonged 'incubation period' in people with Down's syndrome before which symptoms become apparent (Lai & Williams, 1989). These problem areas await further, and perhaps more longitudinal, research for their resolution. However, in view of the publicity given to the link between Down's syndrome and Alzheimer's disease, families and carers may be reassured to know that 'the association of DS and the full clinical-neurological condition of (Alzheimer's) is far from absolute' (Thase 1988, p. 361).

Effect on families

Over the last half century there have been changes in how families of disabled children are seen. In the earlier years they were stigmatised as guilt-ridden, rejecting, and over-protective, often on the basis of no or only flimsy evidence. Later came a greater concern with facts, derived from the views of the families themselves and the problems that they identified, while currently the principal interest is in the coping strengths of the families. In addition there has been a move away from a search for problems (negative outcomes) towards including also the identification of positive outcomes (Sloper *et al.* 1991). Similarly, although 'the family' means more often than not the mother, in some cases attention has also been paid to fathers and sibs. It remains true that the bulk of research concerns families of children with Down's syndrome, with relatively few studies of families of affected adolescents and adults.

In nearly all cases the news that a baby has Down's syndrome comes as a terrible shock† (Berry *et al.* 1981; Ryde-Brandt 1988). Despite this almost

† But not invariably. Six mothers in Carr's (1975) study said the news did not come as a shock to them because they had already discovered it for themselves, or had thought there might be something seriously wrong with the baby, or in one case because the mother already had a child with Down's syndrome.

inevitable distress, much can be done to help the parents cope with it if the occasion is properly managed, the news being given early, sympathetically and truthfully (Cunningham, Morgan & McGucken 1984). The majority of parents (90%) felt they had got over the initial shock within the first month (Cunningham & Sloper 1977). As the child grows older most families adjust and are not seriously impaired. Ryde-Brandt (1988) set out to survey anxiety and depression in mothers of school-age children with Down's syndrome and discovered no differences between them and comparison women who either had a non-disabled child or were childless: only 3/13 of the mothers of Down's syndrome children had scores on the borderline of depression, and none scored beyond that. Van Riper, Ryff & Pridham (1992) found no differences in personal, marital, or family functioning between families with either a Down's syndrome or a non-disabled child. Despite some gloomy pronouncements on the likelihood of marital discord following the birth of a child with Down's syndrome there is little evidence of this (Byrne, Cunningham & Sloper 1988). More marriages were rated poor where the 2 year old had Down's syndrome than in families of non-disabled children but there was no difference in the number rated 'good'; when the two groups were followed up eight to nine years later there were no differences in marriage ratings (Gath 1973; Gath & Gumley 1984). Mothers of children with Down's syndrome went out less often than did those of non-disabled children, both at 15 months and at 4 years old, but expressed themselves as equally content with the situation; 'We go out as much as we want to' (Carr 1975). Sixty per cent of mothers of teenagers in Buckley & Sacks' (1987) study said there were no restrictions on their social life, although almost all of the rest would have liked more choice of leisure and holidays. About a third of the mothers of young adults were working (Holmes 1988; Shepperdson 1992); over half in each case felt their ability to work had been affected by the young person, mainly in the hours they could put in to fit in with the young person's day care, but a much lower proportion, respectively 28% and 39%, felt their husband's working life had been affected in the same way.

Where health was concerned, mothers of 4 year olds with Down's syndrome rated their own health as slightly but not significantly poorer than did mothers of non-disabled controls (Carr 1975). Psychological ill-health was no more common in parents of children with Down's syndrome than in those of non-disabled children (Murdoch & Ogston 1984).

In one of the few studies of older people, mothers of adults with Down's syndrome were more satisfied with their family life and the support services received than were parents of adults with other forms of learning disability (Seltzer, Krauss & Tsunematsu 1993). Looking at the factors associated with stress and satisfaction, mothers of children who were less developmentally advanced and had behaviour problems reported higher stress levels (Hanson & Hanline 1990; Turner *et al.* 1991). Mothers were more likely to be satisfied with life if their child had good self-help skills, but factors unrelated to the child, such as aspects of their own personality, both parents being in employment, and car ownership, also played a large part (Turner *et al.* 1991). Mothers still carry the main burden of care, and this remains true even when the child is disabled and both parents are working (Bristol, Gallagher & Schopler 1987). Generally speaking, fathers show fewer signs of stress than do mothers, and child factors associated with stress for mothers have been shown to be different from those for fathers (Sloper *et al.* 1991). Personality and marital factors were important for fathers, as for the mothers, but financial security was of greater importance for fathers than was employment (Turner *et al.* 1991). Other research (Rodrigue, Morgan & Geffken 1992) has confirmed the extra concern of fathers of children with Down's syndrome about financial security; nevertheless these fathers reported levels of satisfaction, with their parenting and marital roles, which were comparable with those of fathers of non-disabled children.

Not surprisingly, families with other material disadvantages such as poor housing, unemployment and poverty suffer more distress, and these factors had more effect on family happiness than did the factors related to the child (Turner *et al.* 1991). From this it follows that financial and practical help should ease the stress of caring for a disabled child, and indeed this has been shown to be the case (Beresford 1993).

Brothers and sisters

Early studies of the impact of a disabled child on the family suggested that many brothers and sisters were adversely affected (Holt 1958) and that sisters, especially elder sisters, were more likely to suffer (Farber 1959; Fowle 1968). Later research has attempted to confirm these findings and has explored the effects of age and sex (of both index child and sibs), family position, degree of disability, and social class, often comparing families of Down's syndrome children with those of non-disabled children; research methods have been by interview of parents and of the sibs themselves, and direct observation. Overall very few adverse effects have been reported. Sibs neither are reported nor report themselves as overburdened by caregiving (or other) tasks (Boyce, Barnett & Miller 1991; Holmes & Carr 1991; Boyce & Barnett, 1993). They get on well with the disabled sib, and are jealous of him or her to an extent similar to that seen in sibs of non-disabled children (Byrne *et al.* 1988); neither age nor sex has been shown to have a major effect, although in two studies more disturbance was found in sisters (Gath 1973; Cuskelly & Gunn 1993) and especially older sisters (Gath 1974). However, a later study in this latter series could detect no disadvantage to brothers or sisters (Gath & Gumley 1987). Patterns of play between a child and his or her Down's syndrome sib were similar to those between pairs of non-disabled sibs, with the exception that in the Down's syndrome dyads the behaviour of the child with Down's syndrome was comparable to that of second-born children, and that of the sib of first-born children from a normative sample (Abramovitch *et al.* 1987). The conclusion of the authors of the latter study summarises the main thrust of the findings in this area: 'The most striking result is the normality of sibling interaction' (Abramovitch *et al.* 1987).

Overall the main finding of the research concerned with the effect on families has been of 'an overwhelming impression of family "normality", variety and strength' (Byrne *et al.* 1988, p. 135). With all the extra difficulties they face, families of children, and of adults, with Down's syndrome cope, survive, and 'are more comparable to than different from families of non-disabled (children)' (Van Riper *et al.* 1992).

TWO

Populations and procedures

The study originated with all the babies with Down's syndrome born in the year December 1963–November 1964 who lived in the county of Surrey (less the borough of Croydon) and in one area of southeast London (then the boroughs of Camberwell and Lewisham). Fifty-four babies, 25 boys and 29 girls, were referred to and visited by the writer. Forty-five were living at home, nine (three boys and six girls) in various foster homes. Soon after the study began it was decided to include a control group and each home–reared child was matched – for sex, age, and social class – with a non-disabled baby. This sample of non-disabled babies was obtained with the cooperation of the Statistical Division of Somerset House, who, as each baby with Down's syndrome came into the study, supplied names of babies of the requisite sex and social class living within 15 km of the psychologist's home in Surrey. These families were then contacted by their health visitors, who asked for their agreement to a visit from the psychologist. No family refused.

Social class distribution

The family of each home-reared child with Down's syndrome was classified according to the Registrar General's Classification of Occupations (1960) at the outset (age 4) and again at 11 and 21. The distributions at 4, 11 and 21 years are given in Table 2.1.

At age 4 the home-reared children were almost equally divided (49%/ 51%) between middle and working class families, with a slight over-representation of social classes I and II (41%) which was, however, not excessive for Surrey (33%). At age 11 the proportions of middle and working class families were 47%/53%, and at 21, 51%/49%. Figures for the controls were: at age 4, 20 in the middle class and 22 in the working class groups (48%/52%); at age 11, 18 and 19 (49%/51%) and at age 21, 16 and 14 (53%/47%), respectively. For consistency, in analyses that take account of social class the category in which a family was placed at the outset was retained throughout the study. As it turned out, this limitation had little effect. Because of small numbers, analyses by social class were

Table 2.1. *Social class of families of children with Down's syndrome, 4, 11 and 21 (percentages)*

	I	II	III		IV	V
			NM	M		
4 years ($n = 39$)	8	33	8	31	10	10
11 years ($n = 38$)	8	34	5	31	11	11
21 years ($n = 35$)	9	37	5	31	9	9

Definitions used in tables throughout the book: DS, Down's syndrome; M, manual class; NM, non-manual class; N, index child; *n*, number of people; N.A., not asked; N.Ap., not applicable; n.s., not significant; *r*, correlation coefficent.

not carried out using the five major social class groups† but concerned only differences between those in the non-manual (NM) and manual (M) working classes; only one family moved, at 11 years, from the NM to the M category, while one moved at 21 from M to NM.

With sex, age and social class equated between the groups, there were three major factors on which the groups were not matched: size of family, age of the mother, and religion.

The families with a child with Down's syndrome were larger than those of the controls, but apart from a higher proportion of older sibs this difference was not significant. Mean maternal age was considerably higher in the mothers with a baby with Down's syndrome, as was commonly found at that time – 36.6, compared with 28.1 for the controls. These figures are close to those of 35.1 and 28.4 obtained from 2605 mothers of babies with Down's syndrome and controls, respectively (Penrose 1965). In the present study then the mothers of the children with Down's syndrome were on average eight and a half years older than were those of controls. Turning to religious affiliation, just over a quarter of the mothers of the children with Down's syndrome were Roman Catholics compared with only one mother in the control group. These differences, in maternal age and religious affiliation, were each significant at the 0.01 level and have been taken into account in analyses to which they were relevant.

Changes in the populations

Over the years there have been some changes in these populations. The parents of one girl refused further contact after six months; those of

† Non-manual or middle class: groups I, II and IIIA. Manual or working class: groups IIIB, IV and V.

Table 2.2. *Numbers tested and interviewed,*
home- and non-home-reared, and controls
interviewed, at age 4, 11 and 21

	Home		Non-home		Control
	Test	Int.	Test	Int.	Int.
4 years	36[a]	39	6	N.D.	41
11 years	44	43	6	6	38
21 years	41	41	6	6	30

[a] A number of children did not cooperate in testing,
see Carr (1975). Int., interview; N.D., not done.

another emigrated when she was 3; at 11 one child from a middle class
family, a profoundly disabled boy, was seen and tested but as his father
had recently died and his mother was dying the family interview was not
carried out; while at 21 one mother refused permission for the researcher
to visit her 21 year old son because of her anxieties over the confidentiality
of computerised data. Apart from these, all losses from the Down's syndrome group have been caused by deaths. Nine children with Down's syndrome (eight girls and one boy) died before 16 years: two, both girls, by 1
year; three more, two girls and a boy, by 2 years; one girl by 3 years and
another by 7 and two more by 15. One boy in the control group died when
he was 9. Table 2.2 gives the numbers tested and interviews carried out in
both the Down's syndrome and control groups at 4, 11 and 21 years old
(the figures for 6 weeks to 3 years are given by Carr (1975, p. 14)).

Changes also occurred in the families. Three parents of children with
Down's syndrome, two fathers and a mother, died before the child reached
4 years (the deaths of the mother and of one father were accidental), and
a further eight fathers and three mothers by 21 years. Three of the young
people had lost both parents by this time. One father of a boy in the control
group died after the child reached 11. Despite this apparent disparity in
parental deaths between the two groups it has not been possible to show
that this is statistically significant. Three couples out of 45 (7%) in the
Down's syndrome group were divorced by the age 21 survey, compared
with six divorces known to have occurred amongst the 33 control families
(18%) for whom information was available.

There were changes too in the geographical location of the subjects and
their families. Between 6 weeks and 4 years all continued to live within the
original boundaries apart from one child whose family moved to Cornwall
at 6 months and whose parents brought her back regularly for testing in
the author's home. At age 11 six more had moved away (three of them
'non-home-reared' children). At 21 a further seven had moved, making a

total of 13 (32%) who had moved out of the original area, as far afield as
Eire, Somerset, Devon, the West Midlands and Lancashire. Of those controls who could be traced, six had moved away by age 11, one of whom
could not be traced at 21.

Living situation

At the outset 45 children were living in their own homes and nine in non-
home-reared placements, and, apart from the deaths of three non-home-
reared girls, this remained the same at 4 years old. Table 2.3 shows the
living situation for those with Down's syndrome brought up originally in
or out of their own homes, at ages 11 and 21.

By age 11 three of the home boys (including the one whose family
was not interviewed at that time) were in long-stay hospitals; all were
profoundly learning disabled and all the families had severe problems,
of physical or mental illness, in other members of the family. By 21,
five more severely disabled young men and one profoundly disabled
young woman had gone into long-term care. Again the majority of the
families have had major stresses to contend with apart from the Down's
syndrome youngster, but the young people were able to go home regularly at weekends. Two were living in hostels, the young woman from
choice, and the young man because both his parents had died. However,
two girls originally non-home reared were fostered, one at the age of 2
and the other at 7, and though the former, who is profoundly disabled
and whose foster family included a severely learning disabled son, went
into care again at 19 years old, the latter is still and is likely to remain
permanently with her foster family.

Table 2.3. *Living situation, 11 and 21 years, Down's syndrome, home-
and non-home-reared*

| | 11 years | | 21 years | |
	Home	Non-home	Home	Non-home
Own home	34	0	25	0
Foster home	0	2	0	1
Children's home	1	3	0	0
Hospital	3	0	4	0
Residential school/home	0	1	2	4
Private organisation	0	0	2	1
Hostel	0	0	2	0
Total	38	6	35	6

These changes have resulted in over a third (39%) of those with Down's syndrome living away from home at 21. (The figure for those originally brought up at home, 29%, is comparable with the 27% for the controls.) Nevertheless for the purpose of looking at the effect of place of rearing on developmental and other indices, it was decided that it would be inappropriate to include in the out-of-home group those who at later ages were sent to other placements partly, at least, *because* they were very severely disabled. Therefore the children or adults described as 'non-home-reared' comprise only those (six) who left their own families by 6 weeks old.

Testing procedures

Between 6 weeks and 4 years the tests used were the Bayley Infant Scales of Mental and Motor Development (Bayley 1969). The Stanford Binet, form L-M, was used by Bayley to follow on the experimental form of her scales, and this was used for the controls at 36 months (the last occasion on which the controls were tested). The Stanford Binet was attempted also for the children with Down's syndrome, but only one child achieved an IQ at 36 months and five at 48 months, so the scores reported for the children with Down's syndrome were based on the Bayley Scales (Carr 1975).

At age 11 most of the children were given the Merrill–Palmer Scale (1948) and the Reynell Language Scales (Reynell 1969); three profoundly disabled children were given the Bayley Scale of Mental Development in place of the Merrill–Palmer; five were unable to score on the Reynell scales. At age 21 the main assessment instrument was the Leiter International Performance Scale (Leiter 1980). Receptive and expressive language were tested using the British Picture Vocabulary Scale (BPVS) (Dunn *et al.* 1982) and the vocabulary test from the Wechsler Pre-School and Primary Scale of Intelligence (WPPSI) (Wechsler 1967). The equivalent test from the Wechsler Intelligence Scale for Children was attempted but was found to be too difficult for all but six of the most able young women. Reading was tested using the Neale Analysis of Reading Test (Neale 1958) and arithmetic on Vernon's Arithmetic-Mathematics Test (Vernon 1960).

Interviewing procedures

The principal aim of the interviews at the outset of the study was to look at the effect that the young child with Down's syndrome had on his or her family, and, especially, to explore what problems arose beyond those that were likely to occur with any small child. This was made possible by comparison of the responses of two groups of mothers, one with children with Down's syndrome and one with non-disabled children, who were interviewed using semi-structured interview schedules. The schedules were derived, for 15 months, from the 'Guided interview schedule for mothers of children aged one year' (Newson & Newson 1963) and for four years, from the 'Guided interview schedule for mothers of cerebral palsied children' (Hewett 1970), with some alterations to adapt the schedules for use with children with learning disabilities. For the 11 year age group the schedule was expanded to include, by permission, items from the early, experimental version of the Handicaps, Behaviour and Skills (HBS) Schedule (Wing 1980), and at age 21 items used by Holmes (1988) relating to leisure interests and experience of service were also included.

At age 15 months and 4 years the interviews were carried out only for those children in their own homes. This continued to be the case in respect of all those parts of the interview concerned with the other family members – parents and sibs – but at 11 and 21 the parts relating to the individual on self-help and practical skills, personality, friendships, activities and health were discussed also for those living away from home with the principal caregiver concerned.

The interviews were recorded not on tape but in writing by the interviewer, who checked the appropriate categories on the schedules and wrote down verbatim as much as possible of the mothers' replies. Most interviews took about one and a half to two hours to complete but in some cases could last three hours or more. The interviews with the mothers of the children with Down's syndrome and of the controls were carried out in the same way, although there were some questions that were not appropriate to, and not asked of, the mothers of the controls. At 11 years most of the interviews with the mothers of the children with Down's syndrome were carried out by Dr Sheila Hewett (University of London Institute of Psychiatry). Apart from this, all the interviews and tests were carried out by the author.

The nature of the study

This study is individual-cohort based, and is not a multi-cohort longitudinal study (Schaie 1983). The data it contains refer strictly only to those subjects and their families, and those contemporary with them, on whom it is based. Future cohorts have been or will be influenced by circumstances (social, educational and political) that are different from those affecting the population discussed here; hence some caution should be taken in extrapolating the findings to other cohorts.

Symbols and shorthand

To save space here, especially in tables, the groups of those with Down's syndrome and the controls are sometimes designated 'DS' and 'C', respectively; where they are divided into the non-manual and manual worker groups they are designated 'NM' and 'M' respectively. The terms 'learning disability' and 'learning disabled' are shortened to 'disability' and 'disabled'; where any other form of disability is referred to (e.g., physical disability) this is specified in full.

Up to 11 years the subjects of the study are referred to as 'children', males as 'boys' and females as 'girls'; thereafter they are referred to as 'young people' and 'young men' and 'young women', respectively.

All the first names used in quotations from the mothers have been changed.

Unless otherwise stated, significance levels are represented as follows:

* = significant at $P<0.05$ or below

** = significant at $P<0.01$ or below

*** = significant at $P<0.001$ or below

Finally

As before (Carr 1975), it is important to bear in mind that most of the evidence presented here is derived from the mothers' reports and not from direct observation. There is some evidence (Douglas *et al.* 1968) of concordance between observational records of interactions between mothers and their children and the mothers' reports of those interactions given some hours later, so some confidence may be placed in mothers' reports. Much of the data available on child behaviour and family response in families of non-disabled (Newson & Newson 1963, 1968; Thomas, Chess & Birch 1968; Stallard 1993), physically disabled (Burton 1975; Anderson & Clarke 1982), autistic (Wing & Gould 1979; Wolff *et al.* 1989), and learning-disabled children (Friedrich, Wilturner & Cohen 1985; Tunali & Power 1993) has been derived from such reports and, although concerns have been expressed about the accuracy of parental recall of events over time (Chess, Thomas & Birch 1966), this should not similarly affect contemporary reports. Nevertheless the nature of the data should be remembered, and where the reader encounters statements beginning 'so many children did this' or 'so many of the adults did that' it should be understood that they may always be prefixed by 'it was reported that . . .' and taken with a pinch of scientific salt.

THREE

The developmental study

In 1963, at the start of the Surrey study, the task for the psychologist was simply to give developmental tests to the identified cohort of infants with Down's syndrome. Subsequently, the scope of this part of the inquiry was considerably broadened, but the mapping of the intellectual progress of the group has continued to be an important aspect of it. The focus of the intellectual mapping has also broadened: from 6 weeks to 4 years, tests of mental and motor development only were given; at 11 years a test of language was added, and at 21 years tests of academic attainment (reading and arithmetic) were also included. In this chapter the data from the 11 and 21 year studies of intellectual ability (IQ) will be presented, followed by the data on intellectual achievement (language, reading and arithmetic).

Intellectual ability

Results up to 4 years of age, already reported (Carr 1970, 1975), showed that: at 6 weeks old the mean Bayley DIQ of the children with Down's syndrome was significantly below that of the controls; ratio IQs of the children with Down's syndrome declined with increasing age, from a mean of 80 at 6 months to a mean of 45 at 4 years; there was no significant effect of social class, in contrast with the controls; mean scores for girls were significantly higher than those for boys, while those for the home-reared children were significantly above those for the non-home-reared (see Fig. 3.1).

Table 3.1 gives mean IQs at 11 and 21 years for the whole group, and for the group categorised by sex, place of rearing and social class. At 11 years mean IQ for the whole group was 37.2. Girls had a mean IQ more than eight points higher than that of boys but this difference did not quite reach significance. There was virtually no difference between children brought up in or away from their own homes, nor between those from middle and working class families.

By 21 years of age, two young women had died and one young man was withdrawn from the study by his mother. All three came from working class families. When scores for these three are omitted from the

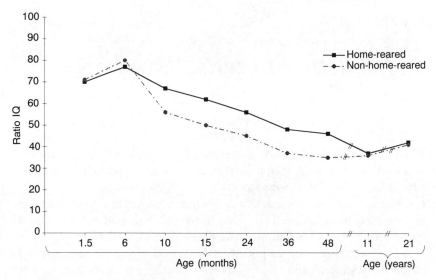

Figure 3.1. Mean IQs between 6 months and 21 years, home- and non-home-reared, Down's syndrome.

Table 3.1. *Means, standard deviations and ranges of 11 and 21 year ratio IQs*

	11 years				21 years			
	n	IQ	SD	Range	*n*	IQ	SD	Range
Whole group	44	37.2	11.9	7–57	41	41.9	16.3	8–67
Males	23	33.2	12.1	7–53	22	37.5	15.8	8–57
Females	21	41.5	10.2	19–57	19	47.0	15.6	8–67
Home	38	37.3	12.1	7–57	35	42.1	16.8	8–67
Non-home	6	36.2	11.3	19–48	6	40.8	14.2	15–57
Non-manual	18	37.1	14.8	7–57	18	38.9	19.8	8–67
Manual	20	37.5	9.5	12–52	17	45.5	12.5	8–59

See Table 2.1 for definitions.

calculations, the 11 year mean IQs for the 41 children present at 21 years increase slightly, by between 0.3 and 0.7, over those for the 44 seen at 11 years, and are as follows:

   whole group = 37.5;

   boys = 33.7;

   girls = 41.7;

   home-reared = 37.6;

   working class = 38.2.

(Ranges were not affected.)

Table 3.2. *Means, standard deviations and ranges of 11 and 21 year mental ages (in months)*

	11 years				21 years			
	n	MA	SD	Range	*n*	MA	SD	Range
All	44	49.9	16.2	9–78	41	59.0	23.6	12–96
Male	23	44.6	16.7	9–71	22	52.8	22.5	12–81
Female	21	55.6	13.9	25–78	19	66.0	23.4	12–96
Home	38	50.0	16.5	9–78	35	59.4	24.1	12–96
Non-home	6	49.3	16.0	35–66	6	56.0	22.5	15–81
NM	18	49.5	20.8	9–78	18	54.5	28.3	12–96
M	20	50.4	11.9	17–66	17	64.6	18.1	12–84

MA, mental age.

At 21 years the mean ratio IQ† showed an increase of 4.7 points (4.4 on the same 41 subjects). As before there was a slight (insignificant) advantage to those from families in the manual group. The previously seen advantage to females had increased, the difference between the raw scores now being significant at less than the 0.4 level. Females predominated in the upper IQ range, males in the lower. For example, over half the females (53%) compared with 18% of the males had IQs of 50+: 10% of the females' and 18% of the males' IQs were below 20. As at 11 years, and in contrast with the results up to 4 years old, there was no significant difference between those brought up within or out of their own homes.

Table 3.2 presents these data in terms of mental ages instead of IQs. (Mental ages from 6 weeks to 4 years can be found in Carr 1975, p. 20). At 11 years the mean mental age was 4 years 2 months (50 months), with a range from 9 to 78 months; at 21 years the mean was 4 years 11 months (59 months), range 12–96 months. From 6 weeks to 4 years mental ages were positively correlated (Carr 1975), although correlations with the earlier tests were low and non-significant. From 10 months onwards correlations rose to between 0.62 and 0.87, reaching 0.92 for that between the 3 and 4 year tests. All were significant at least at the 0.01 level. As is commonly found (Koch, Share & Graliker 1963), correlations between adjacent ages and at later ages tended to be higher.

Correlations between IQs at 11 and 21 years with IQs at all other ages are given in Table 3.3. Correlations up to 15 months were low, confirming

---

† Ratio IQs on the Leiter Scale for subjects over the age of 13 are calculated by the formula: $(MA/13 \times 100) + 5$ (Leiter 1980).

Table 3.3. *Correlations of 11 and 21 year IQs with IQs at all other ages*

	11 years			21 years		
	n	*r*	*P*	*n*	*r*	*P*
1.5 months	24	0.34	0.10	22	0.37	0.09
6 months	36	0.28	0.09	33	0.17	0.33
10 months	40	0.47	0.002	37	0.37	0.02
15 months	41	0.63	0.0001	38	0.53	0.0006
2 years	43	0.72	0.0001	40	0.68	0.0001
3 years	43	0.81	0.0001	41	0.75	0.0001
4 years	42	0.73	0.0001	39	0.68	0.0001
11 years				41	0.90	0.0001

the inadequacy of early infant tests in predicting later development. From 2 years onwards, however, all correlations were significant at the 0.0001 level at least. These results, over periods of between 9 and 19 years in a population with severe learning disability, may be compared with the correlation of 0.75 on tests over a six month period on a non-disabled group, mean chronological age (CA) 12 years (Turner, Mathews & Rachman 1967), although Yule, Gold & Busch (1982) found a higher correlation, 0.86, from a large group of children tested over a longer period at the age of 5 years and again at 16. Nevertheless, the present results support the more usual finding of greater stability of scores in those with learning disabilities (Knobloch & Pasamanick 1960) compared with non-disabled children.

In this population then IQs remained very stable over long periods; tests on groups of children, even in early childhood, predicted with considerable accuracy scores from tests (different from those given earlier) on the same groups in middle childhood and early adulthood. However, as the correlation coefficients indicate, the relationships between the scores at different ages were not perfect, and the scores of some children changed considerably. Figure 3.2 shows the number and magnitude of score changes between 11 and 21 years.

Large score increases of seven points or more from 11 to 21 years were seen mainly (10 out of 16) in the above average young people, while one large decrease (8 points) was also from a young man in this category. However, two large increases, of 12 and 13 points, were from boys scoring well below IQ 30 at 11 years. Apart from the score loss by the able young man just mentioned, and by one previously able young woman, who at 21 years seemed to have been seriously disturbed by the death of her father and was under psychiatric care, all score losses of 3 or more points occurred in the profoundly disabled group.

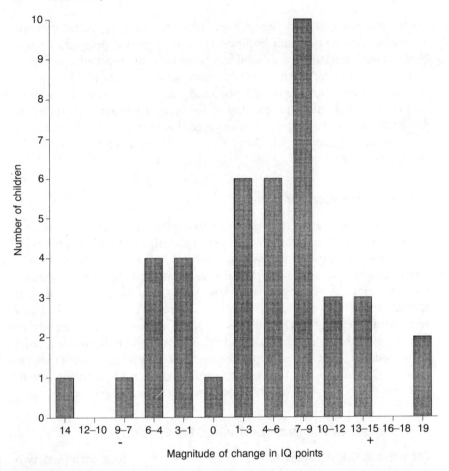

Figure 3.2. Number and magnitude of IQ changes between 11 and 21 years, Down's syndrome.

Correlations with parental education

Some studies have reported IQs in Down's syndrome children to be related to parental IQ and education (Fraser & Sadovnik 1976; Golden & Pashayan 1976; Cunningham 1987), although others have failed to confirm this (Bennett, Sells & Brand 1979; Irwin 1989). In the present study an attempt was made to relate IQ at age 21 to the number of years of education reported by each parent, and to parental education level: a score of 1 represented education no further than secondary school; 2 represented any further training that did not include academic qualifications, and 3 indicated training that included academic qualifications.

Both measures on each parent were correlated with IQ, verbal comprehension and expression, and reading-level score of the offspring at 21 years. None of the correlations was significant and none approached significance except for mothers' years of education and offspring's 21 year IQ ($r = -0.28$, significant at $P<0.06$), reflecting the fact that some of the more severely disabled young people had well-educated mothers. Therefore, in this study there is no support for the suggestion that the IQs and academic achievements of people with Down's syndrome are directly related to the abilities of their parents.

Effects of other variables

Multivariate analyses were undertaken to explore the relative importance of the effects of social class, place of rearing, birth weight, illness, hospitalisation, vision, hearing and weight, parental age at birth, parental education, mother's scores on the Malaise scale, and 'telling' (a score derived from the mothers' descriptions of how well or badly the news of their babies' condition was broken to them). None of these factors had any demonstrable effect on IQ scores except social class at 2 years, the advantage being to the working class children. When previous IQ was added in to the equation, this was shown to be by far the most important predictor of later IQ. So the major factor in predicting IQ from 15 months onwards was previous IQ, and no other factor contributed to any great extent.

The effect of the profoundly disabled group

The present study population contains six subjects (four male and two female), five of whom by 11 and all by 21 years were functioning in the profoundly disabled range. This group, representing 15% of those still in the study at 21, constituted a sizeable proportion of the total cohort. An attempt was made, therefore, to discover whether this group had materially affected the findings concerned with the relationships between IQ and social class, and IQ and parental education, by repeating these analyses omitting this profoundly disabled group. No major changes resulted, and the relationships in question were unaltered. In the present study, although the usual social class effect (Hindley, 1965) was found in the early tests on the control children, no such effect has been found at any stage in the Down's syndrome group. Ability level in this group of subjects appears to be independent of that of their parents. This finding is not isolated (Bennett *et al.* 1979; Irwin 1989). It seems that, when children have Down's syndrome, a consistent pattern of relationships between intellectual level in children and their parents, such as commonly exists in non-disabled populations, cannot be taken for granted.

An analysis was made at each age studied of the IQ scores of two subgroups, defined by the six highest and the six lowest scorers at age 21 (Carr 1992b). There was considerable overlap of individual scores at the early ages, no overlap at 2 and 3 years and none after 4 years. About half the children with very high or low early (10 month) scores continued in those positions. The majority of the remaining subjects had scores that varied somewhat, but five children, two whose scores decreased dramatically and three whose scores increased over time, deserve special mention. The two whose scores decreased, one boy and one girl, both from middle class families, each had very high early scores, the boy being the highest scorer at 6 months and the girl the second highest at 10 months. Their positions in the group then declined: more rapidly for the boy, who was average at 10 and 15 months, and from 3 years onwards was one of the lowest three children in the study; and more gradually for the girl, who dropped to the severely disabled group at 11 years and to the profoundly disabled group at 21 years: she had become phobic and withdrawn at about 9 years old but no other factor could be found to account for this change. The other group of three, a boy and two girls, all brought up out of their own homes, had below average scores from 10 months to 4 years, and then at 11 and 21 years scored at the average level or above. One of the girls was permanently fostered with a family at the age of 7 years, and this might have been thought enough to explain the rise in her scores; but the other two were passed from one (albeit benign) home to another as they grew up. Two points may be made. Firstly, the change in scores and in ordinal position was markedly more pronounced for the two whose scores declined, these going from the top to the bottom of the scores for the whole group, whereas those whose scores increased went only from low to good average. Secondly, no factor could be confidently identified, apart perhaps from the move into a more favourable environment by the girl who was fostered, which could account for these changes.

Clearly the relatively smooth, declining curve obtained by combining IQ scores, such as those of the two extreme groups and indeed of the whole cohort, is not necessarily typical of the progress of individuals. In order to illustrate this the curves of scores of three individuals in each of three groups, those with high, medium and low scores at 10 months, are presented in Fig. 3.3. These data show the variability in the succession of scores gained by individuals with Down's syndrome, and hence, despite the high correlations found in groups over time, how unsafe it is to attempt prediction where individuals are concerned.

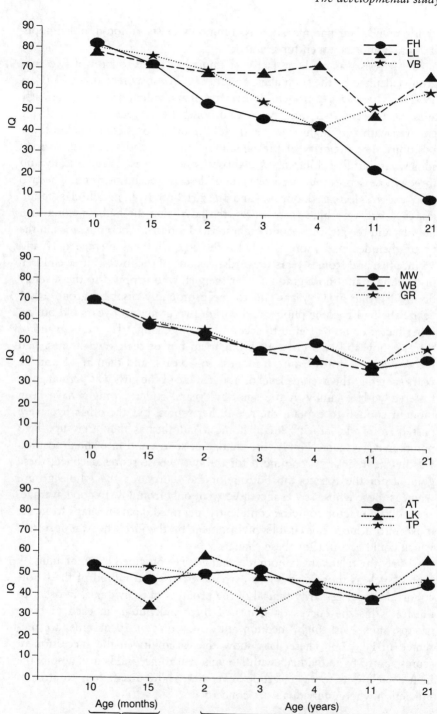

Intellectual achievement

Language skills

At 11 years, all the children with Down's syndrome were given the Reynell Language Scales, comprising tests of comprehension and expression; at 21 years they were again tested on these skills, the BPVS (British Picture Vocabulary Scale) measuring comprehension and the vocabulary test from the WPPSI (Wechsler Pre-School and Primary Scale of Intelligence) measuring expressive language. Table 3.4 gives the results at 11 and Table 3.5 those at 21. At 11 years, Reynell quotients varied between 28 and 38, apart from those for the non-home group which were below 26. At 21 years, mean test ages ranged from 40 to 65 months on the BPVS (comprehension), and from 50 (on a single subject) to 78 months on the WPPSI (expressive) language test.

Reading and arithmetic

At 21 years, reading was tested using the Neale Analysis of Reading Test. Only 16 (two-fifths) of the young people were able to gain reading ages, mean age for accuracy being 7 years 8 months, and that for comprehension 6 years 9 months (see Table 3.6). Two of the most able young women had

Table 3.4. *Means, standard deviations and ranges of Reynell language test quotients, 11 years*

	All (n = 39)	Boys (n = 19)	Girls (n = 20)	Home (n = 33)	Non-home (n = 6)	NM (n = 14)	M (n = 19)
Comprehension							
Mean	32.9	30.7	34.9	34.2	25.7	38.7	30.8
SD	10.5	9.6	11.1	10.4	8.4	11.7	5.8
Range	13–61	16–61	13–60	13–61	16–37	13–61	20–45
Expression							
Mean	33.4	28.1	38.4	35.6*	21.2	41.9	31.0
SD	14.0	9.7	15.7	13.8	7.6	13.2	9.4
Range	8–68	16–63	8–68	13–68	8–28	13–68	19–53

Significance levels used in all tables unless otherwise indicated are: *, $P < 0.05$; **, $P < 0.01$; ***, $P < 0.001$. In this table the subgroups 'home-reared' and 'non-home-reared' were compared. In all other tables significance values are derived from comparing the equivalent data from the Down's syndrome and control groups, unless otherwise stated.

Figure 3.3. IQs of three individuals in each of three groups, those scoring high, medium and low at 10 months, Down's syndrome.

Table 3.5. *Means, standard deviations and ranges of mental ages in months) on language tests, 21 years*

	All	Males	Females	Home	Non-home	NM	M
BPVS							
n	35	18	17	29	6	14	15
Mean	54.0	46.2	62.3	56.9	40.2	65.4**	48.9
SD	20.9	14.5	23.7	20.5	18.4	23.6	16.0
Range	12–111	28–79	12–111	31–111	12–60	12–111	31–83
WPPSI							
n	23	10	13	22	1	11	11
Mean	67.5	56.9	75.7	68.3	50	78.5**	58.1
SD	18.7	9.0	20.3	15.1	0	19.2	11.7
Range	45–105	48–75	45–105	45–105	0	45–105	48–81

BPVS, British Picture Vocabulary Scale; WPPSI, Wechsler Pre-school and Primary Scale. See Table 3.4 for significance level of mean for NM versus M, when IQ allowed for.

reading ages of 12 years 1 month and of 10 years, although they too had comprehension ages which lagged behind, at 8 years 5 months and 8 years 10 months, respectively. Five of the young people, all with reading ages of $7\frac{1}{2}$ or more, were said to read for pleasure – reading books, comics and newspapers: 'and he really reads them, he doesn't just look at the pictures'.

Since the 'floor' of the test, a reading age of 6 years, was too high for the majority of the young people, a 'reading-level' score was also computed to take account of those able at least to name some letters: scores of 1–3 indicated those able to name increasing numbers of letters and 5–9 those with reading ages of between 6 years and 12 years 1 month. Thirty-one young people could be included on the 'reading-level' test as opposed to 16 on reading accuracy. Because almost twice as many subjects contributed to the 'reading-level' score than to reading accuracy the former was often the more useful for statistical analyses.

On the arithmetic test more than two-thirds gained a score (the earliest items on this test consist simply of identifying single numbers). Almost two-thirds (63%) of the young people could do no more on the arithmetic test than recognise numbers and count; ten (24%) could add two figures (e.g. 4+3); seven (17%) could give the number of days in the week; six (15%) could subtract one number from another (e.g. 5–2); three could add money (e.g. four 10p coins and two 5p coins make . . .); only two of the most able could give the number of pence in a pound or do any two-figure adding or subtraction; none succeeded with multiplication or division. The highest arithmetic age, gained by a young man, was 7 years 11 months. Mean

Table 3.6. *Means, standard deviations and ranges of mental ages (in months) on educational tests, 21 years*

	All	Males	Females	Home	Non-home	NM	M
Neale Analysis of Reading							
Accuracy							
n	16	4	12	14	2	9	5
Mean	92.0	86.7	93.0	93.1	84.5	100.4*	79.8
SD	18.8	12.4	20.7	19.9	0.7	14.2	5·6
Range	72–145	72–102	74–145	72–145	84–85	72–145	74–89
Comprehension							
n	14	4	10	12	2	8	4
Mean	81.3	78.2	82.6	82.4	75.0	86.1	75.0
SD	10.0	3.9	11.6	10.5	0.0	11.0	0.0
Range	75–107	75–83	75–107	75–107	0	75–107	0
Vernon's Arithmetic-Mathematics							
n	34	18	16	29	5	13	16
Mean	61.3	58.9	63.9	61.8	58.2	65.2**	59.0
SD	6.9	7.7	4.7	7.1	4.5	8.0	4.9
Range	51–85	51–85	57–73	54–85	51–67	51–85	51–63

See Table 3.4 for significance levels of NM versus M.

arithmetic age was $2\frac{1}{2}$ years behind mean reading accuracy age; this was not simply due to the larger numbers of less able young people included in the arithmetic test because, for those gaining a reading accuracy score, mean arithmetic age was $5\frac{1}{2}$ years, still more than two years below their mean reading age. Even on reading comprehension, where the Down's syndrome people were generally weaker than on accuracy, scores were markedly higher than those for arithmetic: mean arithmetic age for those able to score on comprehension was 66 months, 15 months behind the mean comprehension score.

Test scores and mothers' assessments

The interview with the mothers (or, for those not living at home, with a carer who knew the person well) included questions about reading and number skills, and the responses were rated. Correlations between these ratings and the young people's scores on the attainment tests were high, being 0.77 for the reading level test and 0.70 for number skills, both significant at <0.001. These were very similar to comparable findings by Sloper *et al.* (1990) of correlations of 0.72 and 0.70 between test scores and teachers' ratings of reading and arithmetic, respectively. Reading accuracy and comprehension were more moderately correlated, probably because of small numbers of people;

both correlations were 0.51, significant at <0.05. So those young people with higher test scores tended to be those who were more highly rated; however, relationships between the two assessment methods were not perfect, and even good correlations do not necessarily mean that the actual level of skill indicated by each method was the same. Therefore, if it is of interest to know how people with Down's syndrome compare with others in terms of educational skills, it is essential for standardised instruments to be used.

Correlations

Scores on language, reading level and arithmetic tests at 11 and 21 years were significantly correlated with IQs at all other ages, the correlations from 24 to 48 months being significant at the 0.001 level or better. The exceptions were the scores on the Neale reading ages, which, since the reading level test did reach significance, may have been due to small numbers of people. Correlations between IQ and language and educational tests at 11 and 21 years are shown in Table 3.7. Those who performed better on language, reading and arithmetic were the more able young people, and these results were quite well

Table 3.7. *Correlations between IQs at 11 and 21 years and scores on language and educational tests*

	11 years	21 years
Reynell Comprehension		
r	0.74	
P	0.001	
Reynell Expression		
r	0.73	
P	0.001	
BPVS		
r	0.73	0.65
P	0.007	0.0001
WPPSI		
r	0.64	0.52
P	0.0001	0.003
Reading level		
r	0.71	0.65
P	0.0001	0.0001
Arithmetic		
r	0.67	0.50
P	0.001	0.003

See Table 3.5 for definitions.

predicted by scores on earlier IQ tests. These data do not support the view that there is 'little correlation between achievements in [reading and number skills] and IQ' (Buckley 1985, p. 339).

Correlations between the academic tests themselves were significant at below 0.005 for the BPVS, WPPSI, arithmetic and reading level test ($r = 0.77$–0.56). Reading accuracy was correlated at below 0.001 with the BPVS ($r = 0.77$) and with the reading level test, and reading comprehension at below 0.0001 (0.96 and 0.85).

IQs/MAs for those scoring on achievement tests

Mean IQs, for those scoring on the Reynell scales at 11 years and on the BPVS at 21 years, are only slightly above the general means because all, but a small minority with severe disabilities (six at each age), were able to score on these tests. On the academic tests at 21 years, a larger proportion could not attempt the tests, so mean IQs and MAs for those who could are higher than the general mean. All these data are shown in Table 3.8. For those able to score on the BPVS and WPPSI, mean Leiter mental age was 64.7 and 71 months, respectively, compared with mean test ages of 54 and 67.5 months, respectively, for those tests (see Table 3.5). Thus, verbal ages were 10.5 and 3.5 months below the Leiter ages, showing that in this group verbal skills were less advanced than general ability. This also lends support to the view that the increase in IQ seen in this group at 21 years may be due to the absence of verbal items in the IQ test used.

Table 3.5 shows that mean age on the test of receptive language (BPVS) was lower than that of expressive language (WPPSI), partly because of the larger number of the less able young people who were able to score on the

Table 3.8. *Means IQs and mental ages (in months), and ranges of mental ages for those children with Down's syndrome able to score on language and educational tests*

	n	IQ	MA	Range
Reynell				
Comprehension and Expression	39	39.9	53.8	25–78
BPVS	35	45.9	64.7	12–96
WPPSI	23	50.2	71.0	33–96
Reading				
Comprehension	14	54.3	76.9	63–96
Accuracy	16	54.0	76.5	63–96
Arithmetic	34	48.1	68.0	51–96

See Table 3.2 and 3.5 for definitions.

BPVS. However, the mean BPVS age of those able to score on the WPPSI is 65 months, leaving the mean expressive language age still $2\frac{1}{2}$ months ahead. On the Reynell scales too there was little difference between the two scales, with expressive language slightly ahead (see Table 3.4). There is no evidence from this study, therefore, to support Cornwell's (1974) suggestion that the verbal deficit in children with Down's syndrome can be attributed to a particular difficulty in verbal expression.

On the arithmetic test the mean test age of 61.3 months (see Table 3.6) is seven months behind the mean MA for this group, but in contrast with this finding, and with those on language, mean ages on the reading tests are above their respective Leiter ages, reading comprehension being four and reading accuracy 15 months ahead. So as a group the Down's syndrome young people were doing less well on arithmetic but better on reading, and especially on reading accuracy, than would be expected from their mental ages.

If we look at scores for individuals, 26% had arithmetic ages that were equal to or above their Leiter MAs, but in respect of reading accuracy this was true for 81% of individuals. Ten young people had reading ages which were 10 months or more higher than their Leiter MA; the highest, in a young woman, being 49 months higher than her Leiter MA (which was itself the highest of the whole group). Those with higher arithmetic ages were mainly the less able young people; all except one had below average Leiter MAs and only that one (the young man with the highest arithmetic score) made any score on the reading test, while, with the exception of that young man, none could do more on the arithmetic test than recognise numbers and count. So those with higher arithmetic than Leiter ages were those with quite limited skills overall who had, nevertheless, learned some, very elementary, arithmetical processes.

Group differences in ability and achievement

Differences by sex

At both ages (11 and 21) mean scores on intelligence tests of the females were higher, and the difference on raw scores was significant at 21 years. On achievement tests scores of the females were higher in every case, but the differences were not significant after allowance had been made for IQ.

Differences between home- and non-home-reared

At neither 11 nor 21 years was there any significant difference between scores on intelligence tests. At 11, the home-reared children had significantly higher scores on the expressive language scale, even after controlling for IQ. At 21, although scores for the home-reared were higher in every case, the differences were not significant when IQ was allowed for.

Differences by social class

Intelligence test scores of those in the working class (M) group were higher than those in the middle class (NM) group but these differences did not reach significance. In contrast, on achievement tests the scores of the young people from the NM group were superior in all cases, and this superiority was significant, after allowing for IQ, at the 0.05 level for the Reynell expressive language test, and at below the 0.03 level for both 21 year language tests and for arithmetic and reading level, while for reading accuracy the difference was significant at the 0.05 level. Trends for the 11 year Reynell comprehension, and for 21 year reading comprehension were in the same direction, favouring the home-reared, the women and those from NM families, but the differences were not significant.

Discussion

Intellectual ability

Studies of intelligence in children with Down's syndrome have commonly found IQs to decline with increasing age (Melyn & White 1973; Ludlow & Allen 1979; Morgan 1979) or, less commonly, to remain relatively stable (Kostrzewski 1974; Schnell 1984). Where increases have been found in the teenage years these have been on very small numbers, of four or fewer subjects (e.g. Cornwell & Birch 1969; Connolly 1978). The decline has been variously suggested as resulting from deterioration of cerebral function, artifacts of test construction or content, or specific neuromotor and sensory disabilities emerging with age, but no definitive conclusion has been reached (see Gibson 1978, pp. 30–34).

In the present study mean scores declined until 11 years, so the mean increase at 21 years, of nearly five IQ points, was unexpected. The population remained substantially the same, with only two losses between ages 11 and 21, subtraction of the scores of these two from the 11 year mean resulting in an increase of only 0.2 points. So the increase in mean IQ at 21 does not appear to be due to the loss of low-scoring subjects, and the 21 year mean is similar to that reported from a group with an average chronological age (CA) of 28 (Holmes & Carr 1991). Berry *et al.* (1984) present results from 28 adults aged between 15 and 42 years, mean CA = 21, who gained a mean MA of $5\frac{1}{2}$ on Raven's Coloured Progressive Matrices. This corresponds exactly to the 21 year mean MA in the Surrey sample discussed here, excluding the six profoundly disabled young people who would not have been able to attempt Raven's test. Six years later, mean MA in the Berry *et al.* (1984) study rose from $5\frac{1}{2}$ to $7\frac{1}{2}$ years, more than twice the increase seen from 11 to 21 years in Surrey. However, unlike in Surrey, this two year gain was achieved on identical tests. Although the possible remedial effects of the programme in which the group was involved must be taken into account, it appears that a real gain may have been demonstrated.

Correlations between IQs over time were high (see Table 3.3), especially at the later ages, representing considerable 'constancy of ordinal position' (Clarke & Clarke 1984). As Clarke & Clarke (1984) point out, even high correlation coefficients do not guarantee stability for all members of a population: in the present case, seven young people (17%) showed IQ changes at 21 years of more than 10 points (six upwards), four of these (10%) by 15 or more points. Clearly then, despite the stability of the group, and although the proportion of large score changes (over 10 points) is lower than the near 30% found by Tew & Laurence (1983), dogmatic prediction of the future developmental level of any individual with Down's syndrome would be unwise.

Much of the early work on the mental development of children with Down's syndrome was concerned with the differences between those brought up either within or out of their own homes (Dameron 1963; Shotwell & Shipe 1964; Stedman & Eichorn 1964; Shipe & Shotwell 1965; Bayley, Rhodes & Gooch 1966). All showed the home-reared children to be at an advantage, and this was also the case in the early stages in Surrey. At 11 years, however, and again at 21 years, no difference could be seen in non-verbal IQs, although there was a suggestion of some superiority in language for those brought up at home. It should be remembered that the non-home-reared Surrey children were not brought up in large institutions but in small homes and foster homes, and almost certainly received a great deal more individual attention than was previously possible for the institution-reared children. Nevertheless, although the effect on verbal skills still needs to be explored further, the effect of in-home rearing on non-verbal IQ may be less pronounced in the long term than it was in the early ages. Even this finding may soon be only of historic and academic interest, as babies with Down's syndrome who cannot remain in their own homes are welcomed into adoptive families.

Those studies that have looked at sex differences in the intelligence of children with Down's syndrome have shown scores of females to be higher (Clements *et al.* 1976; Connolly 1978; Gath & Gumley 1984; Schnell 1984; Cunningham 1987). Gibson (1978, p. 104) suggests that this difference is due to selective mortality, the more severely disabled females dying earlier, and this conjecture would be compatible with the relative paucity of severely disabled females in the present study. During the course of the present study eight girls (and one boy) died, and the mean IQs of the girls, from 1.5 months onwards, were compared with those of the girls who survived. At 1.5 and 10 months the means of the girls who subsequently died were eight and nine points, respectively, behind those of the survivors, but at all other ages the scores were within four points of each other, and at 4 years were slightly higher for those who died. Therefore, in this study there is little support for the hypothesis that the higher scores of females are due to selective mortality, although it remains possible that they may be due to differences in mortality before 6 weeks old. The hypothesis would not explain the excess of high scoring girls, and this still awaits explanation, but as this finding has not been remarked on in other studies it may be due to chance factors.

Others have pointed to the greater linguistic facility of females as an explanation for these differences between the sexes (Schnell 1984; Cunningham, 1987). Cunningham (1987, p. 175) proposes that this 'may not be some inherent factor but related to interactional style within families', paralleling ideas put forward about the same phenomenon in non-disabled children (Newson & Newson 1977, p. 186). This hypothesis deserves exploration. In Surrey the difference between the scores of the sexes increased steadily over the years and was largest at age 21, when the test used required no language, and when the females' superiority on tests of language was not significant when allowance was made for IQ: the 'language-superiority' hypothesis was not supported here. No study, so far as is known, has shown males with Down's syndrome to be of superior intelligence. As Gibson (1978, p. 108) has already indicated, the possibility must be entertained that female sex confers some advantage to populations with Down's syndrome.

In Surrey, neither social class nor parental education was associated with IQ. Cunningham (1987) found both factors to be significantly associated with child mental age, parents of higher social class and with higher educational levels having children with higher mental ages. In Surrey, despite the use of similar measures of social class and parental education, the direction of the effects, although not significant, was the reverse of that seen by Cunningham, with slight advantages to children and adults from working class families. Two possible explanations of these differences between the two studies were considered: firstly, the presence in the Surrey sample of a quite large proportion (15%) of profoundly disabled young people, and, secondly, the much smaller size of the Surrey sample. The profoundly disabled young people came mainly (4 out of 6) from middle class homes, so relationships of IQ with parental education and social class were recalculated, omitting these subjects. This resulted in a slight shift towards the positive end of the scale, correlations of IQ with parental education going from between −0.37 and 0.025 to between −0.18 and 0.012, but all remained very small and insignificant. The second consideration was whether the difference might be due to differences in size between the two studies: the Manchester group is roughly four times bigger than its Surrey counterpart. However, the numbers in the latter are similar to those in other studies in which positive relationships with parental abilities have been reported (Fraser & Sadovnik 1976). Although larger numbers may have resulted in associations more like those found in Manchester, nothing in the figures as they stand suggests that this is likely to be the case. It may be that such findings will not be seen invariably and that populations of people with Down's syndrome, like individuals within such a population, will vary considerably one from another.

Intellectual achievement

People with Down's syndrome are known to have particular difficulty with speech (Gibson 1978, p. 234; Fowler 1990), although not necessarily with communication, and with academic tasks, number work being as a rule more delayed than reading (Wallin 1944; Kostrzewski 1965, cited in Gibson 1978, p. 182; Cornwell 1974; Irwin 1989). Data on academic skills are, however, sparse. Reading is often reported only in terms of the number of words read (Lorenz, Sloper & Cunningham 1985) and there are few reports of reading tests and reading ages. Some individual high achievers are described, with reading ages of 9 or 10 (Butterfield 1961; Duffen 1976; Buckley 1985), but only three reports of group data have been traced. Pototzky & Grigg (1942) give results for nine young people, mean CA 20, mean IQ 55, whose mean score on the Monroe Silent Reading Test was about $8\frac{1}{2}$ years. Dunsdon, Carter & Huntley (1960) used Burt's Reading Accuracy Test with eight children, mean CA 11, mean IQ 54, and obtained a mean reading age of 8 years 8 months. In a study from McQuarie University (Pieterse & Treloar 1981) eight children, who had been in an early intervention programme and had gone on to ordinary schools, at a mean age of 8 and with a mean Stanford Binet IQ of 59, had a mean reading age of 7.2 years. This is close to the mean reading age of 7 years 8 months of the 16 young people in the present study (mean IQ 54).

Data on arithmetical skills are even fewer. An 11 year old has been said to be able to do long multiplication and to add and subtract five-figure numbers, with or without a calculator (Duffen 1976). Of 5 year olds at McQuarie, only one had reached the level of adding one or two to a single digit, and all the eight children in normal school were bottom of their class for number work, although only three were bottom of the class for reading. In Pototzky & Grigg's (1942) sample of 20 year olds, 50% could perform simple addition and 30% three-place addition and subtraction; 35% 'knew their multiplication tables' and 50% were said to be able to do long multiplication (though Gibson finds these figures 'difficult to credit' (Gibson 1978, p. 182)). The group studied by Dunsdon *et al.* (1960) were given Burt's Oral-Arithmetic test, resulting in a mean arithmetic age of $4\frac{1}{2}$ years, 4 years behind their average reading age.

Against these reports of academic achievement those of the present cohort seem unimpressive, being lower than Pototzky & Grigg's (1942) on number work and not much better than the McQuarie 8 year olds on reading. Three points may, however, be relevant: firstly, results in the present study were obtained from all those in an unselected population who were capable of any reading or number work, and not, as seems likely in some other studies, from highly selected populations; secondly, in the present study scores are based on formal, one-off testing, whereas in some studies the levels reported may have been attained on a number of different informal occasions; and thirdly, in the present study, the young people had been out of full-time education for 3–5 years, while in other studies they were still in school or in continuing education.

Data from all the studies reviewed here have shown people with Down's syndrome to develop better reading than arithmetical skills. It is pertinent to inquire whether this is a characteristic of the syndrome, or whether it is typical of people with learning disabilities generally. A study of children with spina bifida (Carr, Pearson & Halliwell 1983) showed that children without any disability had number ages that were commensurate with their reading ages, as had the controls, while those with disabilities, including lower IQ, had number ages which were 7–11 months lower than their reading ages, although the gap between reading and arithmetic did not widen as IQ decreased. Children with spina bifida may constitute a special group, since their learning disability is due to a known cause, the effects of hydrocephalus. In the case of non-specific learning disability, Kirk (1964) cites a number of early studies, most (11 out of 14) showing 'mentally retarded' children in special classes to read at levels below that expected from their mental ages (*ibid.* p. 73); and (*ibid.* p. 81) that in arithmetic they achieved at expected levels in 'arithmetic fundamentals' (presumably addition, subtraction, division and multiplication), citing one study that found this population to score higher on arithmetic fundamentals than on any other school subject (Witty & McCafferty 1930). However, in arithmetical reasoning scores were lower (up to 24 months lower) than would be expected. None of the young people with Down's syndrome in Surrey attempted anything beyond the fundamental arithmetical tasks, so the pattern of scores in children with non-specific learning disability reviewed by Kirk (1964), that is reading scores below and arithmetic scores above expected levels, is the opposite of that commonly found in people with Down's syndrome. However, in a more recent, though small-scale, study (Rutter, Tizard & Whitmore 1970), learning-disabled children in the Isle of Wight, mean IQ 68, had arithmetic scores somewhat lower than those for reading, being 1.7 standard deviations below the mean for the controls, compared with 1.2 standard deviations below for reading.

Level of IQ may be important: in none of the studies discussed, of children with non-specific learning disability, was the IQ as low as that in the Surrey group. It might be that if a group with non-specific disability and IQs similar to those in Surrey were investigated, their abilities would be found to have patterns similar to those of people with Down's syndrome (although higher IQ did not, in the Surrey group, reverse the trend; of the nine 21 year olds with the highest IQs, ranging from 57 to 67, all had reading ages that were above and arithmetic ages that were below their mental ages).

The position is, therefore, not clear, although with all studies of people with Down's syndrome showing them to do better at reading, and most studies of other populations of people with learning disabilities showing them to do better in arithmetic, it may indicate a difference in skills between people with learning disabilities of different aetiologies. The resolution of this discussion awaits controlled studies carried out on matched groups.

Females in the present study had higher scores than males, as has been shown elsewhere (Jones & Casey 1990; Sloper *et al.* 1990). However, this difference disappeared when IQ had been allowed for: this factor was not considered in the Jones & Casey (1990) study, and did not alter the position in that of Sloper *et al.* (1990), where the assessment of academic skill relied on checklist ratings by teachers. Nevertheless social class, which did not feature significantly in the Sloper *et al.* (1990) study, was significant in the Surrey group, with those from professional and managerial backgrounds surpassing those from manual workers' families; and this difference was still significant after controlling for IQ.

These findings were the more unexpected as there were no parallel findings on IQ. Nevertheless, where verbal and academic skills are concerned, there appeared to be clear environmental effects, with the young people from more advantaged backgrounds doing significantly better than those from the less advantaged. Although at 21 years no measure was taken of how much deliberate teaching the parents were doing, visiting the homes did not give the impression that any were spending much time on this. The influences at work seem likely to have been the more subtle ones of atmosphere and expectations, of availability of relevant materials – books, magazines, newspapers – of modelling of skills by other family members and opportunities to join in with these activities. However this may be, the indications support Buckley's (1985) view that 'people with Down's syndrome can progress to levels of academic skill which would not have been thought probable. In 1978, Gibson suggested that 'Many DS children are exposed to traditional academic training simply because it has parent status value' and 'the outcome is frequently an increase in stress levels for the child and a decline in self-regard without any useful educational gain.' In the present study, it has been clear that for some, at least, of the young people attainment of good reading skills has contributed to their self-confidence and given them a source of real recreational pleasure. It seems important that schools which currently *are* teaching children with Down's syndrome to read (Lorenz *et al.* 1985) should not be discouraged from doing so since even quite limited literacy can contribute to greater independence and enjoyment in adult life.

FOUR

Self-care and independence

The degree to which a child or adult can take the responsibility for looking after his or her own personal needs can have a major effect on the burden of care for the family, and on the person's own sense of independence. These skills were not, in the Surrey study, observed directly, but were reported by the parent (usually the mother) or principal caregiver in the course of structured interviews carried out at 15 months and 4, 11, and 21 years. This chapter focusses on: 1, sleep and mobility; 2, the four major areas of feeding, washing, dressing and toileting; 3, coping with puberty; 4, achievement in the four major areas combined; and finally at the relationships between the four major areas as shown by correlations.

Sleep and mobility

At the earliest ages (15 months and 4 years) the Down's syndrome children slept as well as did the non-disabled children (Carr 1975) and this pattern of reasonably good sleep routines continued, three-quarters of the children in both the Down's syndrome and control groups, and four-fifths of the adults with Down's syndrome sleeping well. Ten of the children in each group and nine of the adults with Down's syndrome would wake early in the morning or be very late going to sleep at night (Table 4.1). In the children with Down's syndrome this behaviour could be problematic: one

Table 4.1. *Sleep at 4, 11, and 21 years, Down's syndrome (percentages)*

	4 years (n = 39)	11 years (n = 43)	21 years (n = 41)
Slept well	77	68	78
Needed attention	23	16	22
Had nightmares	0	19	15
Late sleeper/early waker	0	23	22

See Table 2.1 for definitions.

boy regularly woke early, following which he would rampage through the house strewing things around, tipping over and smashing others, and he could only be coped with by locking him in his room. By 21 years no such strategy was necessary for him, and none of the other 11 year old late sleepers/early wakers now disturbed the household.

Eight children and nine adults with Down's syndrome needed some attention at night. For one mother this meant only that she put on the light by her bed when her 21 year old son needed to go to the toilet, but for others more was demanded of them.

11 years

She sleeps in my room, I'm afraid she'll choke when she's sick, I wouldn't let her have a room of her own yet. I get up to her two to three times every night. It's a continual source of worry.

He likes to be up at six o'clock in the morning to put on his records. I get so tired when he is at home, his poor sleep is the reason he lives away from home.

21 years

He'll wake up and get up and put on his music very loudly. If we took his tape recorder away he would only go and find ours, or he'd find *something*, the TV or video. We have to get him back to bed very quickly and then he goes to sleep again.

He cries and shouts out when he has a nightmare about mum's death, and I have to sit with him. We can have three or four of these a week or a week will go by without his having one, but he is always a light sleeper. [This young man has lived permanently with his sister and her family since his widowed mother died, when he had been the one to find her dead in bed.]

Eight children (and five controls) and six adults with Down's syndrome sometimes had nightmares. Two children with Down's syndrome, who could not talk, were presumed to have nightmares when they cried out in their sleep, while for another her mother was uncertain whether what she had was a nightmare or a fit. One girl with Down's syndrome and one control boy, but none of the adults, sometimes walked in their sleep.

Where mobility is concerned, all the children and young people could walk, and 91% of the children and 71% of the adults with Down's syndrome could run at least 45 metres. At 11 years, three out of the four who could not run were profoundly disabled boys who walked stiffly and could not manage stairs well (in one case not at all), but the fourth was a capable girl with heart problems who had good walking

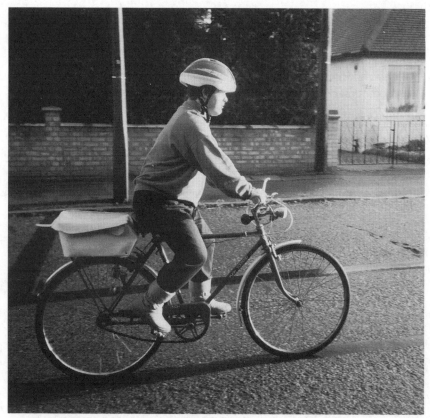

Model cyclist

skills, although she could not run. At 21 years, eight who ran at 11 now no longer did so; five of these had significant heart problems and the other three were considerably overweight. One profoundly disabled young man now ran, but one similarly disabled young woman, who ran at age 11, no longer did so. Two-thirds of the children rode tricycles well and with enthusiasm; four, two boys and two girls, were competent bicyclists. By 21 years, five were cyclists, only one of these having been so at 11 (this young man was well known in his town for his cycling skills and had been commended for them by the police – 'if everyone rode their cycles like he does we wouldn't have any trouble'). However, of the three other 11 year old cyclists, one girl had died and one young man's mother had refused further contact, leaving only one young woman who was known to have given up cycling.

Self-help skills

Feeding

Table 4.2 shows that at 11 and 21 years all could feed themselves, over half the children and four-fifths of the adults managing independently (about half and a tenth, respectively, of these needing help with difficult foods, for example bones in fish). Another third of the children, but only three adults, who used a knife and fork, could not always cut tough foods. Six children and five adults still ate with a spoon; three and four, respectively, were profoundly disabled, most of the remainder being in the severely disabled group apart from one boy who at 11 years had a persistent feeding problem. The large majority ate a normal diet but four at 11 years had a liquidised diet and seven at 21 years had their food chopped, minced or mashed; all were severely or profoundly disabled apart from the boy with the feeding problem just mentioned. He had been on a liquidised diet at home throughout his school life, refusing anything lumpy, and his mother had not known that for most of this time he had eaten ordinary school dinners, learning this only after he had been at the adult day centre for 18 months. Since then he had been on a normal diet also at home ('meat, lumps, everything, he chews it all up'), had graduated to independent use of a knife and fork, and his feeding problem was largely resolved. Two children needed help in drinking and one of these, a profoundly mentally and physically disabled young man, still needed help at 21. Five at 11 years and four at 21 dribbled but three of those who had dribbled at 11 no longer did so at 21. Nearly a third of the children and half the young people were faddy about at least some foods, although in only one case

Table 4.2. *Feeding at 4, 11, and 21 years, Down's syndrome (percentages)*

	4 years (n = 39)	11 years (n = 43)	21 years (n = 41)
Uses spoon	69	14	12
Uses knife and fork, with help	0	32	7
Eats independently, helped with difficult foods	0	26	10
Eats independently, no help	0	28	71
Eats a normal diet	77	91	83
Drinks alone	77	93	98
Dribbles	N.A.	12	10
Has food fads	N.A.	30	49

at each age (and not the same one) was this a problem. Three-quarters of the young people had impeccable table manners and over four-fifths could cope well if taken out for a meal. Seven (five of the profoundly and two of the severely disabled group) were poor, messy feeders who could not be taken out without embarrassment, though not always because of their table manners.

> It's her burping – she cleared McDonalds once.

Washing

Nearly half the children and two-thirds of the adults could bath themselves without help, the majority of these children and all the adults drying themselves as well (see Table 4.3). Seven adults still needed help in bathing.

> [*How much can she bath herself?*] It's a moot point. I let her bath herself but she doesn't do it properly. She always has a sore bottom, back and front, and she scratches herself. Every two or three days I give her a good going over.

Five at 11 years and four at 21, all profoundly disabled, had to be washed. Three at 21 years were the same profoundly disabled young people as at 11 (and one was the young man not seen at that time), but two of this group had made progress, one very sick young man being able to wash his hands and face and one young woman to bath herself with help. Two-thirds brushed their teeth without help, but hair washing could be done by less than a third (seven men and five women). Two-fifths could dry their own hair using a towel (12%) or a hair drier (29%) while a further 17%

Table 4.3. *Washing at 11, and 21 years, Down's syndrome (percentages)*

	11 years ($n = 43$)	21 years ($n = 41$)
Is washed	12	10
Washes own hands, face	21	10
Baths, with help	21	17
Baths, without help	16	0
Baths and dries, without help	30	63
Brushes teeth, with help	39	22
Brushes teeth, without help	49	68
Washes hair independently	N.A.	29
Dries own hair	N.A.	41

were said to have hair which could be left to dry, making a total of 58% who needed no help with hair drying.

Dressing

A third of the children and two-thirds of the adults dressed themselves without help, two-thirds of these in each case selecting the clothes they would wear (see Table 4.4).

21 years

If he's going out he makes himself very smart. He puts on a collar and tie, sometimes a bow tie. He takes a pride in his appearance and quite fancies himself. If he's going to a dance he'll dress up for it.

Over a third of the children needed some help, with laces, buttons and tight or difficult clothing but by 21 years two-thirds could manage all buttons, and only the profoundly disabled group were not able to manage any. Over four-fifths of the children could undress themselves and nearly half (45%) brushed their own hair, and these proportions were virtually identical in the adults.

Toileting

Three-fifths of the children and two-thirds of the adults were reliably clean and dry by day, around a quarter more had only the occasional accident (see Table 4.5). At 11 years two of the boys could not urinate standing up and on outings their mothers took them with them to the 'Ladies' – 'So far no one has objected'. For one mother, toileting was 'the problem of

Table 4.4. *Dressing at 4, 11, and 21 years, Down's syndrome (percentages)*

	4 years (n = 39)	11 years (n = 43)	21 years (n = 41)
Dressed	58	5	2
Much help needed	24	23	15
Some help	16	39	17
No help	2	33	66
Undresses, without help	N.A.	82	83
Cannot manage buttons	N.A.	N.A.	15
Manages all buttons	N.A.	N.A.	66
Brushes own hair	N.A.	45	46

Table 4.5. *Toilet at 4, 11, and 21 years, Down's syndrome (percentages)*

	4 years (n = 39)	11 years (n = 43)	21 years (n = 41)
Day			
Doubly incontinent	8	9	5
Sent to toilet	N.A.	5	7
Takes self, occasional accident	N.A.	26	20
Reliably clean and dry	38	60	68
Cleans self after toileting			
with supervision	N.A.	25	20
no supervision	N.A.	55	66
Night			
Doubly incontinent	8	9	7
Enuretic	59	14	10
Dry if lifted	15	7	2
Clean and dry	18	70	81

my life', as her son had, after his father's death and following a stay in short-term care in hospital, regressed from being clean and dry. Another mother had given up trying to toilet-train her profoundly disabled son when he became 9 years old. Half and two-thirds, respectively, could clean themselves after using the toilet and about another quarter could do so with some supervision. The six, who at 21 years were not able to clean themselves, comprised two very severely and four profoundly disabled young people, but one profoundly disabled girl managed independently and one with some help.

Over two-thirds at 11 years and over four-fifths at 21 were dry at night. Of those not dry at 11, one was a very capable girl who it was felt was given rather little opportunity by her family to develop her self-care skills. Another was a boy with numerous compulsive traits who also had a considerable toileting problem – he refused to use any toilet except the one in his family home. Soon after the interview at 11 years he was taken into a special unit, where one of the tasks undertaken was to teach him to generalise his toileting skills. This was successfully accomplished and the family wrote a triumphant postcard: 'We have taken him for the day to Southampton and he used a Southampton toilet!' At 21 years he was unreliable about toileting, although his general abilities were average for the group.

Coping with puberty

Females

Mean menarcheal age as reported by the mothers was $13\frac{1}{2}$ years (for two of the young women in care it was not known). Three of the girls had started their periods at the age of 11, four after they were 16, one of these at 19 ('I thought she wasn't going to and perhaps she had no womb'). Fifteen, 79%, had very regular periods. Only a third had trouble free periods, the remainder suffering at least some pain and four suffering quite severely. Twelve of the 19 young women (63%) coped independently with their periods, assembling everything they needed, changing and disposing of their pads, and if necessary washing out stained knickers. Four of those who were not independent in this were the four most severely disabled young women, but three were young women in the middle range of ability. Just over half had no mood disturbance at the time of their periods but six were liable to be irritable and two, one of whom was also irritable and weepy, became more lethargic at this time.

Males

Mean age of attaining puberty for the boys, as reported by their mothers, was 14 years. Two boys had become pubertal at 12 years old and four had not become pubertal until 17 or 18. One profoundly disabled young man was not yet pubertal. Six of the 22 young men could not shave themselves at all; five of these were profoundly or severely disabled but one was a quite able, but rather unpredictable, young man. Two, one of them the profoundly disabled young man not yet pubertal, did not yet need to shave. A battery operated razor was used in all except one case ('He only needs shaving once a fortnight and he doesn't like the noise of an electric razor so we use a safety'), but only nine (41%) of the young men were able to shave themselves independently. One young man was solving the problem by growing a beard.

Total independence

An independence score was computed comprising: feeding (feeds self, eats normal diet, drinks alone); washing (washes, baths and dries self, cleans teeth, washes and dries hair); dressing (dresses, including managing fastenings, undresses self); and toileting (clean and dry by day, and by day and

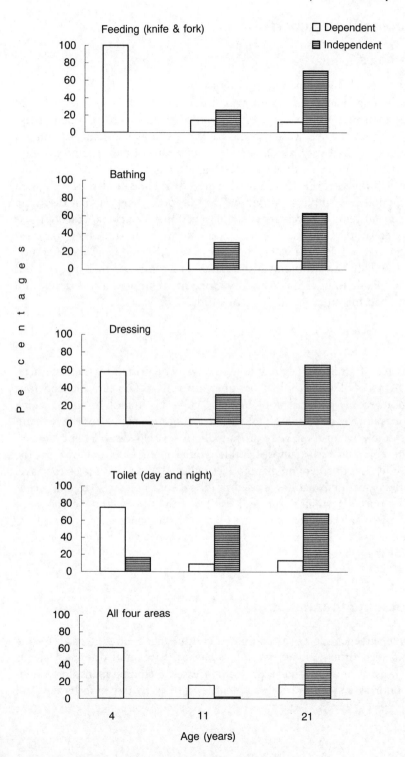

night, cleans self). Figure 4.1 indicates the proportions of those independent and totally dependent at 4, 11 and 21 years. After 4 years of age, those totally dependent were very severely and profoundly disabled individuals.

Fairly steady progress was made over the years, most between 4 and 11 years, although further progress was still possible beyond that age. However, at 11 years only two children, one boy and one girl (the latter having been in care all her life) were fully independent, although a quarter needed very little help. Seven children, including the boy with compulsive behaviours, were very dependent, but one profoundly disabled girl who had been in care all her life did not fall into this group.

At 21 years over two-fifths (44%) were fully independent. Six young people, including the young man not seen at 11 years and the one with compulsive behaviours, were still very dependent but two who had been very dependent at 11 years (one of them a young man with a heart defect who died shortly after the interview) had mastered sufficient skills to be able to manage in most areas, albeit with some help. Where full independence had not been achieved, bathing was the main difficulty for nearly half (49%), problems with hair washing accounting for most of that.

Correlations

Correlations at each age of each self-help score with the other scores, at ages 11 and 21, showed that at 11 years dressing skills were significantly related to those of feeding and washing, and these were related to each other; total independence was highly significantly related to feeding, washing and dressing, but toileting was not related to any other score. At 21 years all skills, including toileting, were strongly related to each other (see Table 4.6)

Longitudinal aspects

The two main factors considered in attempting to predict competence in self-help were IQ and previous self-help scores. IQs at 2, 3, 4, 11 and 21 years were each correlated with the self-help score at ages 11 and 21 (see Table 4.7). At 11 years all previous IQs were significantly related to total independence but, where individual skills were concerned, only washing was related to IQs at 3 and 4 years, dressing to IQ at 3. No previous IQ

Figure 4.1. Proportions of young people independent and totally dependent at 4, 11 and 21 years, Down's syndrome.

Table 4.6. *Correlations (r) of self-help scores at 11 and 21 years,*
Down's syndrome

	Feed	Wash	Dress	Toilet
11 years				
Wash	0.49*			
Dress	0.52**	0.43*		
Toilet	0.07	0.22	0.17	
Total independence	0.72***	0.81***	0.74***	0.29
21 years				
Wash	0.74***			
Dress	0.70***	0.74***		
Toilet	0.71***	0.79***	0.86***	
Total independence	0.76***	0.94***	0.84***	0.84***

Significance levels are indicated as follows:
   * = $P < 0.01$
  ** = $P < 0.001$
 *** = $P < 0.0001$

Table 4.7. *Correlations (r) of self-help scores at age 11 and 21, Down's*
syndrome, with IQs at 2, 3, 4, 11, and 21 years

	IQ at year:				
	2	3	4	11	21
Self-help, 11 years					
Feed	0.17	0.30	0.15	0.43*	
Wash	0.31	0.45*	0.46*	0.57**	
Dress	0.36	0.45*	0.24	0.54**	
Toilet	0.11	0.22	0.18	0.27	
Total independence	0.44*	0.56**	0.44*	0.70***	
Self-help, 21 years					
Feed	0.53**	0.66***	0.49*	0.78***	0.72***
Wash	0.53**	0.55**	0.44*	0.65***	0.61**
Dress	0.43*	0.51**	0.43*	0.60***	0.67***
Toilet	0.43*	0.54**	0.44*	0.63***	0.64***
Total independence	0.49*	0.54**	0.42*	0.62***	0.64***

See Table 4.6 for significance levels.

was related to feeding or toileting at 11 years. At 21 years, IQs at all the previous ages were significantly related to all areas, reaching 0.85 in the case of total independence, similar to the figure of 0.80 reported by Ross (1971).

When regression analysis was used to explain the scores at 4 years, IQ at age 3 had some effect on scores for feeding and night-time continence, but even with the addition of sex and social class these account for less than 23% of the variance, and IQ had no perceptible effect on total independence. At 11 years, total independence was quite well accounted for by IQ at age 4 (42%) and this was hardly added to by the inclusion of sex and social class. Substituting the 4 year independence score for the 4 year IQ gave a much reduced percentage, less than 10%, but using 11 year IQ in place of either independence or IQ at age 4 resulted in a dramatic improvement, with 77% of the variance now accounted for. So at 4 years, IQ had much greater predictive power than independence at that time, and total independence at age 11 could be largely accounted for by the 11 year IQ.

At 21 years, total independence was well explained by the 11 year IQ (65%), and sex and social class added only another 4%. Using IQ at 21 years in place of that at 11 increased the proportion explained by only 9% but substituting independence at 11 years increased this to 85%. Of the individual skills at 21 years, IQ at 11 made the greatest contribution to all except self-management at the toilet, which was more influenced by the same factor at 11. With IQ allowed for, no effect could be seen of sex or social class but those young people brought up from infancy out of their own homes had higher mean scores for dressing and total independence.

In general, neither sex nor social class had any demonstrable effect on self-help skills, either singly or in combination. Total independence was difficult to explain at age 4, but was predominantly influenced at age 11 by IQ and at age 21 by previous levels of independence. It seems that the timing of the acquisition of these skills may be quite variable in young children, so that the level they achieve by the middle school years is little related to their achievements in the pre-school years and is more closely governed by their innate ability. By middle school age, however, the pattern of the children's skills is more clearly defined, and this, although it is still strongly associated with ability level, predicts with considerable accuracy the level of independence they will achieve as young adults.

Discussion

The number of young people who had limited skills in each of the skill areas remained fairly constant from 11 to 21 years. These, as has been suggested earlier, were on the whole the profoundly and very severely disabled young people who, if they had not acquired skills by age 11, were able to make little further progress over the next ten years (although some did make some small gains). Apart from this very disabled group, considerable gains were made in eating, washing and dressing by the remainder of the cohort so that by 21 years the proportion who coped well with these had roughly doubled. The exception was toileting which showed little change, either by day or by night, in the skills attained. This may have been at least partly because a quite high level was reached by 11 years – three-fifths were dry at 11, compared with one-third or fewer with comparable levels of skill in feeding, washing and dressing. It may be that, since toileting is such an essential accomplishment both practically and socially, families and teachers put a special effort into this, while a lesser degree of competence in the other areas is tolerated.

These data from the Surrey study may be compared with those from three other studies that have included examination of self-help skills in young people with Down's syndrome: those by Buckley & Sacks (1987), Holmes (1988), and Shepperdson (1992). Buckley & Sacks (1987) obtained questionnaire data from the parents of 46 children aged 11–14 and 44 adolescents aged 14–17. Shepperdson (1992) interviewed the parents and carers of 53 adolescents aged 14–17 and followed them up nine years later as young adults. Holmes (1988) interviewed parents and carers of 41 young people, mean age 28, half living at home and half in residential care. Each researcher inquired about feeding, bathing, dressing and toileting. Table 4.8 gives the percentages of those said to be fully independent in each area for each of the three studies (figures are given for the older group only in the studies of Buckley & Sacks and of Shepperdson); figures from the Surrey study are also shown for comparison.

Bearing in mind the differences in the populations, survey methods, and possibly also in the definitions of 'independent', the figures are quite similar across the four studies, apart from the lower figures given by Holmes (1988) and Shepperdson (1992) for dressing and bathing. Buckley & Sacks (1987) present figures that are generally the highest of the four surveys; as their group was the youngest (some ten years younger than those seen by Holmes and Shepperdson), this is surprising. The explanation may lie in the different survey methods used. The Buckley & Sacks data were gathered by means of a questionnaire filled in by the parents, while those of the three other surveys by means of interviews: it may be that when parents are interviewed, and probing questions are used to elucidate any answers that are unclear, the criteria are more strictly adhered to, whereas when parents themselves fill in questionnaires they have some latitude in being more optimistic in their responses.

Table 4.8. *Percentages Down's syndrome young people fully independent at age 21 in Hampshire (1), Wales (2), London (3) and Surrey (4)*

	Geographical area of study			
	1	2	3	4
Eating	75	62	58	71
Bathing	68	46	41	63
Dressing	75	33	36	66
Toilet				
Day	84	60	78	68
Night	95	77	88	81

Areas: 1, Hampshire – Buckley & Sacks (1987); 2, Wales – Shepperdson (1992); 3, London – Holmes (1988); 4, Surrey – Carr, discussed here.

Taken together, the studies show that children growing up with Down's syndrome acquire many of the same skills as do non-disabled children, but they acquire them more slowly; in the case of some individuals it seems uncertain whether they will ever acquire all the skills that would enable them to be fully independent. Even as young adults, between a half and a quarter were not fully independent in each individual area, apart from toileting where somewhat higher levels of skill are seen. In the Surrey study most skills were in place by 11 years, and Shepperdson (1992), the only other researcher to have followed up the same group into adulthood, also noted that minimal progress, especially in toileting, was made between adolescence and adulthood. Taking the four skill areas together, less than half the Surrey group were able to look after their own self-care entirely, and Holmes (1988) gives an even lower figure of 5% with this degree of overall competence. Even in adulthood, and notwithstanding the minority who become skilled and self-reliant, a sizable proportion of people with Down's syndrome continue to need supervision or practical help in the daily tasks of their own self-care.

Although in Surrey the self-help scores of the females were slightly higher, no study has found sex to be a significant factor where these skills are concerned. It may be that the self-help areas under consideration are so basic that there can be no question of their being seen as more appropriate to one or the other sex; all need to be as self-reliant as possible, both to enhance their own feelings of competence and independence and to maximise their ability to function in and to be accepted by society. It is interesting to speculate how these skills may best be taught to people with Down's syndrome. The indication in Surrey of a minor advantage to the young people who grew up out of their own homes (supported by similar results given by Holmes (1988)) suggests that, if parents are not on hand to help, the young people may be better able to develop their skills. Berger & Cunningham (1983) show that infants' vocal and social skills blossomed when their mothers allowed them more time to respond, rather than rushing in with help and stimulation. It might be that a similar approach to self-help teaching, with parents and care-givers keeping a lower profile, would pay dividends in this area too. This remains a matter for future researchers to determine.

A major finding in the present study has been of the importance of IQ, and this adds to the weight of similar findings from other studies (Ross 1971; Gath 1985a; Holmes 1988; Turner *et al.* 1991). There is agreement that measured intelligence *is* relevant to the capability of people with Down's syndrome in their daily lives; self-help skills, like academic skills, are more easily acquired by the able than by the less able children, although other factors, such as the opportunities and encouragement provided, were seen in individual cases to have been important.

In other researches, levels of self-help skills in people with Down's syndrome have been compared with those in matched groups of people with learning disabilities of other aetiologies: those with Down's syndrome have been found to be the more competent (Silverstein *et al.* 1985), and this has been seen to be true especially for the groups with severe and profound disabilities (Zigman *et al.* 1989). Silverstein *et al.* (1985) discount the possibility that this is yet another result of the Down's syndrome stereotype, of people with Down's syndrome being particularly favourably rated, since behaviours rather than 'abstract personality traits' were measured; instead they hypothesise that the stereotype may have had an effect on the service providers, mediating their behaviour and enabling them to elicit more positive behaviour from their clients with Down's syndrome. This, as the authors say, is speculation, and it would repay investigation, but the finding appears well grounded: it seems that, for whatever reason, people with Down's syndrome are able to make better use of their abilities in practical matters of daily life than are others with similar abilities. This will have important implications for people with Down's syndrome, who should be well placed to develop to the maximum the skills that will enable them to live independent lives in the normal community.

FIVE

Behaviour and discipline

Intellectual level and the degree of intellectual disability, while of great importance, are not the only matters of concern to the parents of a Down's syndrome child: of almost equal concern are the child's temperament and amenability, how he or she fits in with the family and gets on with other people. We asked mothers about the child's personality and behaviour, behaviour problems, habits and fears, and how the mothers tried to manage these.

Personality and manageability

At each age the mothers of both groups were asked to rate their children's personality, their willingness to cooperate with reasonable requests and how easy they were to manage. The results are shown in Table 5.1. Most parents of both groups saw their offspring as having happy, easy going personalities. More than half the Down's syndrome 11 year olds were described as 'affectionate', 'lovable', 'nice' and 'getting on well with people' (as were 44% of the controls). Other positive descriptions included 'placid' (9%), 'cheerful' (9%), and 'generous', 'sensitive' and 'fun'. At 21 years these terms were applied to 34% of the Down's syndrome youngsters, and other terms now included 'thoughtful', 'interesting', 'more grown up', 'fun' and 'funny'. Four more were described as 'likeable' (these tended to be the more disabled young people). Six mothers at 11 years and nine at 21 years spontaneously described their youngsters as stubborn.

Most mothers had positive comments to make, although some also had reservations.

POSITIVE

11 years

He's very easy going he's cheerful, teases people and has a laugh. He's really quick-witted and loves anything involving a play on words.

She's very nice, a happy child. She's determined and tries hard at school, but she is aware of her limitations.

Table 5.1. *Personality, cooperation and manageability, 11 and 21 years, Down's syndrome and controls (percentages)*

	DS		Control	
	11 years	21 years	11 years	21 years
Personality				
Happy, no adverse comment	56	32	39	50
Happy, some adverse comment	39	58	47	37
Only adverse comment	5	10	14	13
Cooperativeness				
Usually agrees with requests	37	56	41	57
Varies	49	39	43	23
Usually objects	14	5	16	20
Manageability				
Easy to manage	56	76	62	70
Fairly easy	35	17	16	17
Not easy	9	7	22	13

See Table 2.1 for definitions.

21 years

He's very pleasant, always cheerful and friendly, everyone is his friend. He makes friends wherever he goes and he makes them for me too.

She's lovely; if she's away we miss her terribly.

RESERVATIONS
11 years

She's very affectionate, a nice child though she can be stubborn. She knows other children and goes to their houses, but she can't keep up with them so they don't always want her. It's very nerve-wracking; I haven't had a moment's peace with her.

He's a horror! It's difficult to say really; he's good company and nice to take out, and his speech is good so he chats to us.

21 years

People like her; she always gets a crowd round her. She's slightly over friendly and childish; she wants to cuddle people. It was all right when she was younger, people found it endearing, but now it can be a bit embarrassing.

He's like he always was. I love him and hate him. When he's good; he's lovely.

Table 5.2. *Aloofness, 11 and 21 years, Down's syndrome (percentages)*

	11 years	21 years
Aloof and indifferent	2	7
Responds, does not initiate contact	26	12
Makes appropriate social contact	72	81

Two mothers at 11 years and four at 21 years could not find anything good to say.

11 years

She can be moody and she's naughty at times, though she goes very quiet and humble. If she's upset she can be really nasty.

21 years

She's rather anti-social just now, she is not as tactful as she was. I feel people who don't know her or know about handicap may dislike her; I'm afraid they're going to think 'Oh, she's a nasty girl.'

So most of the Down's syndrome group were seen as having easy, pleasant personalities, and most made appropriate social relationships. However, one at 11 years and three at 21, all profoundly disabled young men, were said to be habitually aloof and indifferent to people (Wing & Gould 1979) (see Table 5.2). A further four boys and six girls at 11 years, and two men and six women at 21 years were said to be aloof occasionally, half and all but one, respectively, being profoundly or severely disabled. The exception at 21 years, a young woman of above average ability who had been disturbed by the death of her father, featured at both ages, as did also the three profoundly disabled young men. Altogether at 21 years just under 20% of this population were described as aloof, compared with 38% of the population of a longstay mental handicap hospital (Shah, Holmes & Wing 1982).

Manageability

In both groups there was a general tendency towards the young people becoming more agreeable and easier to deal with as they got older (see Table 6.1). At 11 years, just over one-third and at 21 years just over half were usually cooperative, and nearly half variable, these figures being very similar in both the Down's syndrome and control groups. The six who at age 11 would usually balk at anything they were asked to do, had IQs in the average to low average range, but by age 21 only two, both profoundly disabled, were similarly described.

Not surprisingly, the majority of those who were cooperative were also found easy to manage, both at age 11 (Down's syndrome 75%, controls 93%) and at age 21 (Down's syndrome 96%, controls 89%), but many of those whose cooperation was more variable were also said to be easy enough to manage (at age 11, Down's syndrome 55%, controls 44%; at age 21, 62% and 66%, respectively). Almost all those described as stubborn were seen as easily managed, only two (at 21) as variable. It appears, that it is not necessarily the initial negative response to requests that is crucial, but rather how far parents can be successful in modifying them.

11 years

He's a lot easier now, more reasonable, you can explain things to him and he's not so unpredictable. In many way he's a sensible child.

We all give in to him more than to the others but he gets smacked if he's naughty; he knows how far he can go.

21 years

She's got her own point of view but she will be guided by me. I say, 'I'm older than you and more experienced'. We chat an awful lot.

He's easy enough to manage as long as you treat him as grown up. He's very conscious of the fact that he's grown up.

Understandably the problems seen by the two groups of mothers, those in the Down's syndrome and those in the control groups, were different. For the controls, problems were mainly connected with being self-opinionated, moody or rebellious (although in some cases these traits were seen as having a positive side): for those with Down's syndrome, at 11 years they tended to be destructive, difficult in company and demanding, while at 21 years problems of cooperativeness or management were concentrated in those with severe and profound disabilities, who continued to be stubborn and resistant, and were more difficult to manage now they were bigger.

Fears

Over half the children were afraid of something (Down's syndrome 58%, controls 62%). In the Down's syndrome group this was mainly of dogs (19%), spiders, moths and birds (9%), the dark (14%) and noises (7%), while one child was afraid of dying, another of blood and two more of water, these figures being very similar to those given by Buckley & Sacks (1987) for their teenage sample. In the controls, four were frightened of the dark, three of moths and spiders, three of dying and two of noises, but other fears in this group concerned anxieties about such factors as school work and sport, medical procedures and family matters.

At 21 years two-thirds of the Down's syndrome young people (66%) had fears of some kind, again mainly of dogs and, sometimes, also of cats (22%). Fear of the death of one or both parents occurred in five (12%); in three cases the fear was of the possibility of the parent dying but in two the fears centred around the death of a parent which had already occurred. Four (10%) were afraid of flies, spiders or snakes, four of rain, thunder, wind and/or the dark, and four, all rather frail, severely disabled young people, showed fear when they felt themselves to be physically insecure. Three were afraid of noises, and two of medical or dental procedures.

At age 21, mothers of the controls were not asked about fears, but nearly two-thirds (61%) were said to be worriers, 'mainly about small things', e.g. work, money, exams. These mothers still felt themselves in close touch with this part of their son or daughter's life, almost four-fifths (79%) saying they felt they knew about the worries that he or she had.

Habits

Table 5.3 shows that at age 11, one-third of both the children with Down's syndrome and the controls bit their nails or sucked their thumbs, or both. None of the controls but just over a quarter of the children with Down's syndrome (four boys and eight girls), were said to masturbate, and by 21 years this had increased to one-third (32%), although now only three very handicapped young people did this in public. It seems probable that when they were younger the controls were more careful to do this privately, and in adulthood those with Down's syndrome had in the main learned to be similarly circumspect. A quarter (22%) of the 11 year olds with Down's syn-

Table 5.3. *Habits age 11, Down's syndrome and controls, age 21, Down's syndrome (percentages)*

	DS		Controls
	11 years	21 years	11 years
Bites nails, sucks thumb	39	N.A.	38
Rocks	22	34	0
Masturbates	28	32	0
Self injures	15	15	0

drome and a third (34%) of the adults were said to rock, although in each case half would do so only occasionally. Tongue protrusion, however, was a rarity, mentioned by only three mothers at 21 years, five more commenting that the young person had done this in the past but had learnt not to do so.

Head banging too was unusual, shown by two at age 11 and one at age 21 (and four more adults were said to have done so previously and to have given it up). Five at each age showed some other form of self-injury – picking at finger and toe nails, face smacking, pushing teeth until they bled – but none of this amounted to a serious problem, except in the case of two profoundly disabled young men who at 21 years scratched their own faces severely and frequently.

We asked the mothers what they did about these habits. At 11 years only a quarter of the mothers in each group would try to stop the children from carrying out their habitual actions, the rest either calling the child's attention to it (Down's syndrome 52%, controls 36%), or doing nothing at all but hoping the child would grow out of it (Down's syndrome 29%, controls 41%). There was then very little difference in the reactions of the two groups of mothers, despite the fact that for the controls their habits consisted only of thumb-sucking, nail-biting and nose-picking, while for the Down's syndrome children they included also masturbation, rocking and some self-injury.

By age 21, nine mothers of young people with Down's syndrome were trying, or had in the past tried, to stop their offspring masturbating; three had had some success in that the young person was thought to do this now only in private (as did 11 others for whom no action had been taken), but repeated efforts had been made in the cases of the three who still masturbated in public. Nine mothers had tried to stop their children rocking (one of these had also taken action on masturbation) but none had been entirely successful. Of the ten children who had rocked at age 11, one had died and eight of the rest were among the 14 said to rock at 21.

Altogether at 11 years, nearly three-quarters (72%) of the children with Down's syndrome and over half (59%) of the controls displayed at least one habit, and by 21 this had declined in the Down's syndrome group to under a half (44%). Nearly half of these showed the habit frequently, whenever they had nothing else to do, and this included all the profoundly disabled young people. Those whose habit was infrequent had ability levels over most of the range, only the most able and the profoundly disabled young people being unrepresented here.

Specific behaviour problems

In the Down's syndrome group behaviour problems specifically asked about at each age were aggressiveness, rebelliousness, pestering for atten-

Table 5.4. *Behaviour problems, 11 and 21 years, Down's syndrome (percentages)*

	11 years	21 years
Aggressive	21	19
Rebellious	49(9)	68(5)
Pesters for attention	35(2)	27(10)
Temper tantrums	30	25(5)
Problem behaviour in public	34(8)	22(2)
Multiple problems		
Two	35	32
Three	16	7
Four	2	2
No problems	14	19

Figures in brackets denote the proportion (%) in whom the problem was more than occasional or minor (these figures are contained also in the main percentage figures).

tion, temper tantrums and difficult behaviour in public. The percentages of those showing these problems are given in Table 5.4. Around a third of the children and one-fifth to a quarter of the young adults showed each problem, apart from rebelliousness, which was seen in about half at age 11 and in over two-thirds at 21. As indicated in the table, the large majority of these problems were thought of as quite minor. For example, 'aggression' mostly meant bossiness, bad temper, and occasional swearing, although one girl at 11 years and one young man at 21 years were said to have been rough in the past, while one (delightful) young man had recently 'gone mad' and broken a door when his brother stopped him from going to the pub. Again, two at 11 years and one at 21 years (all severely or profoundly disabled males) were too difficult to take out in public but the problems with the remainder consisted mostly of minor difficulties in shops – taking things off the shelves, talking too loudly or being over-friendly to all and sundry. One boy, who had been extremely difficult as a small child, as an 11 year old could be taken to the supermarket and would put things in the trolley ('not always what you want') and at age 21 'takes your arm and walks like a gentleman'. Therefore, for most parents of adults these problems were not having a major impact on their daily lives.

Six children and eight adults showed none of these problems, these being in each case evenly distributed over the social groups (NHR, non-home-reared)

11 years: NM = 17%, M = 10%, NHR = 17%;
21 years: NM = 17%, M = 29%, NHR = 17%,

and clustering in the mid- to upper ability range (IQ 40–57) apart from one profoundly disabled young man at 21 years. Twenty-three children and 17 adults had two or more problem behaviours: of these seven children and three adults had three while one had four problem behaviours at both 11 and 21. Those with single and multiple problems were represented over the full range of abilities; boys were slightly more likely to be rebellious (boys = 14, girls = 8) and young men to have tantrums (men = 7, women = 3), while females were more likely to pester for attention (girls = 9, boys = 6; women = 8, men = 3). In this study therefore sex, social class and ability level were not clearly related to behaviour problems, although more able children were somewhat more likely to be problem-free and less likely to have multiple problems.

Comparing these figures with those from other studies, Buckley & Sacks (1987) also found about 30% of their under-14 year olds having temper tantrums, though in the Byrne *et al.* (1988) study, of 2–10 year olds, the figure was only 4%; while only 20% in that study were attention seeking compared with the 35% shown in Table 5.4.

Serious trouble

Few in the controls and very few in the Down's syndrome group had been in real trouble at school, with neighbours or with the police (see Table 5.5.). Only five children with Down's syndrome (12%) were said ever to steal, compared with 12 (32%) of the controls. Other troublemaking, at school or with neighbours or the police, was extremely rare, affecting only two children (5%) compared with six controls (16%). These two Down's syndrome children were of average ability: the boy had been in trouble briefly at school for tearing up a cardboard pig, the girl for 'fighting and biting' at school and for vaguely described trouble with the neighbours.

> She has done things, throwing things over the fence and things like that, but they give her a lot of leeway.

With the controls too the trouble was mainly minor but two children had been cautioned by police for shoplifting, and one of these also for causing damage on a caravan site.

Table 5.5. *Trouble at school, with neighbours, and with police, 11 and 21 years, Down's syndrome and controls (percentages)*

	DS		Controls	
	11 years	21 years	11 years	21 years
Trouble at school	4	N.Ap.	11	N.Ap.
Trouble with neighbours	2	0	3	7
Trouble with police	0	5	3	13

At age 21 two young men with Down's syndrome, both of good ability, had been in trouble with the police. In one case there had been a rather 'fuzzy' incident involving stone-throwing at a youth club, and uncertainty as to whether the young man with Down's syndrome, had really been implicated. In the other a young man had been involved in two misunderstandings with girls; the police were called but no further action was taken. Six of the controls (20%) had been involved in some incident, three concerning motoring offences, but none resulting in custodial sentences.

Discipline

Parents have to cope with difficult behaviour, attempting to control and, if possible, improve it. We asked the mothers what methods they used: whether they used punishment for misdemeanours and whether they used rewards (see Table 5.6). In both groups of 11 year olds some children were still smacked but this was markedly more frequent for those with Down's syndrome, where nearly three-quarters, compared with less than a third of the controls, were smacked at least once a month by their mothers (significant at $P <0.01$). The difference in the proportions of fathers who smacked was similar (24% Downs syndrome, 5% controls), but not significant. Looking at individual behaviours, there was a minor and non-significant tendency for the mothers of those rated as rebellious to use more smacking: mean smacking scores at age 11 were 2.2 for those rated as rebellious and 1.6 for non-rebels, and at age 21 were 1.9 and 1.6, respectively. Since at any age rebels may be more likely to be smacked than non-rebels, the smacking of each of these groups at 11 years was related to rebelliousness at age 21. In each group, of those who were and those who were not rebellious at 11 years, more who had been smacked once a month or more were rebellious at 21. In view of small numbers the figures were combined, showing that 55% of those smacked rarely or never were rated

Table 5.6. *Disciplinary methods, age 11, Down's syndrome and controls (percentages)*

	DS	Control
Mother smacks, 1+ per month	71***	30
Threatens	18	19
Deprives (sweets, TV)	31	57*
Dismisses (out of room, etc.)	21	54**
Uses rewards	61	76

See Table 3.4 for significance levels.

Table 5.7. *Disciplinary methods, age 21, Down's syndrome and controls (percentages)*

	DS	Control
Persuade, bargain	58	17
Insist, prompt, compel	22	8
Scold, punish, threaten	15	4
Ignore, leave it	5	17
Give viewpoint, let N decide	0	54
Uses rewards	41	0

as rebellious at 21 compared with 77% of those smacked once a month or more. The difference between the groups is not significant so can be seen only as a trend.

Both groups of parents used other methods as well, which may be grouped under three main headings: deprivation, threats and dismissal. Depriving the children of sweets or TV occurred in both groups, of pocket money only in the controls; in all cases the proportion using these methods was higher in the controls. Overall, significantly more mothers of controls used deprivation and dismissal (sending to bed *etc.*) as punishments. It may be that by 11 years, the more sophisticated disciplinary measures used by the parents of the controls were thought by the parents of the Down's syndrome children to be beyond their children's comprehension, and that they would be more likely to understand the immediacy of a smack. However, threats, to send the child away or of an authority figure (teacher, policeman), and rewards, were almost equally used, by less than a fifth and by over two-fifths, respectively, of both groups of parents.

At age 21, when we asked the mothers what they did if the young person refused to do something he or she really had to do, the methods they used had changed somewhat, as seen in Table 5.7. At this time most mothers of the Down's syndrome young people used persuasion, bargaining, explanation, reasoning and giving the young person plenty of time. One mother described what she called her 'low cunning' approach whereby, when her daughter balked at something, usually a shopping expedition, she would 'turn it to her advantage' by suggesting they include in the expedition the purchase of something her daughter particularly wanted. Many mothers emphasised that it was 'no good having a head on collision'. Only 11 mothers ever used any form of punishment, mainly deprivation of some possession such as books or tapes, but one young man would be kept in, another had his hand smacked and another, profoundly disabled, young woman would be made to sit in a particular chair following a misdemeanour. Five mothers would speak firmly or insist on the required behaviour and four more, especially of those young people who were still small and physically manageable, would supplement this, where necessary, with physical prompting. Two would ignore any refusal to co-operate, saying that the young person would come round eventually to their point of view.

In contrast, less than a fifth of the mothers of the 21 year old controls would try to persuade their young people into cooperation. Over half would not attempt this at all, but would put their point of view and then leave it to the young person to decide what action he or she would take. These mothers had confidence in the judgement of their son or daughter, which was not, on the whole, shared by the mothers of the Down's syndrome young people.

None of the disciplinary methods used by the mothers at 11 or 21 years was related to the children's behaviour at the time; that is, no significant difference was seen in the use of either punishments or rewards between offspring who had or did not have behaviour problems, nor between those found to be more or less cooperative or easy to manage, although, as might be expected, there was a tendency for those who were easier to manage to be punished less. It may be that parents use these methods either on principle or at random, since there is little evidence for their effectiveness.

Longitudinal aspects

Aspects of behaviour, 11 to 21 years

Some categories of fears featured at both ages – dogs, flies and spiders, the dark, wind and rain, and noise – but there was very little consistency in an individual's fears from one age to another. Only four who had feared dogs and one who had feared spiders as 11 year olds still feared these at 21.

Half of the surviving eight young people said to be aggressive at age 11 were said to be so also at age 21, although now only occasionally. However, two-thirds (65%) of those rebellious at 11 years were found to be the same at 21 years, and only four (20%) were never rebellious at this time. Almost half (45%) continued to have tantrums. Of those who had pestered for attention at age 11, 60% continued to do so, and constituted two-thirds (7/11) of those pestering at 21. Three of the 16 showing difficult behaviours in public at age 11 still did so at 21 (19%), in all but one this being only a minor problem.

So nearly half the young people having temper tantrums at 11 years continued to do so as 21 year olds, and half continued to be aggressive to some degree, although an equal number of those not showing these behaviours at the earlier age had developed them later. Just over half who were difficult to take out in public at age 11 were still so at 21. However, if young people did not pester, rebel or show difficult behaviour in public at age 11, it was unlikely they would show these behaviours at 21.

Habits

Four young people of the ten surviving to age 21 who were known to have masturbated at 11 (40%) were still known to do so, three being severely or profoundly disabled and the fourth with average ability. Two of the original 12 had died but the remaining six were no longer said to masturbate. However, nine young people who had not been identified at 11 years were now said to masturbate, all but one doing so privately, and a further two were said to have done so in the past, although they had had not been identified at age 11. So in this group masturbation once begun was not necessarily established for good, and could begin at different stages in life; in adults in the upper-severe range of ability or above (IQ 30+), it was likely to be done, perfectly appropriately, in private.

Of the nine surviving children who had rocked at 11 years one no longer did so at 21 years. A further six young people now rocked who had not done so at 11 years. Those still rocking (and indeed those rocking now but not at 11) tended to cluster in the below-average ability range, apart from one young woman of above average ability. Rocking then seems likely to persist from childhood, but may also begin later when it has been absent in the early years. Only six children (14%) were said at age 11 to injure themselves, and in none was the injury serious. At age 21 two of these were still doing so and the injury (self-scratching) was now more severe and frequent. Five more, not identified at 11, were said to have shown some self-injurious behaviour (in four, head banging) in the past but this had disappeared. Of the five ever said to bang their heads, this behaviour persisted to a minor degree in one, led on to severe alternative self-injury in two more, minor alternative self-injury in the fourth, and had disappeared in the fifth. Of the 11 (one-quarter of the total) who had at any time showed any self-injury, some form of the behaviour persisted to some degree in six (14%) and had disappeared in the remaining five. In this population self-injury, especially head banging, tended to be minor and short-lived, but if self-injurious behaviour persisted, as in this case in two profoundly disabled young men, it was relatively severe.

Corbett (1975) concludes that mild self-injurious behaviour occurred in 5–15% of severely retarded people, was more common and severe in younger people, and severe self-injurious behaviour requiring symptomatic treatment was much less frequent than milder forms of the behaviour. This is supported in the Surrey group in whom mild self-injurious behaviour occurred in seven (16%) of the 11 year olds, and five (12%) of the 21 year olds. In none of these (including the two young men who scratched themselves) did the scale of the injury meet Corbett's criterion of severity, that of requiring symptomatic treatment. In this group, then, mild self-injury occurred at a rate consistent with that found in other populations of people with severe handicaps, but self-injury of sufficient seriousness to require treatment was absent.

Early discipline and later outcome

We looked at how the methods used by the mothers to regulate their children's behaviour related to the behaviours the children showed at later ages. We considered, at 15 months, and 4 and 11 years, how the mothers reported that they supervised their children, their use of a variety of punishments and rewards (Table 5.8); at 4 and 11 years, of parental attitudes to discipline and the parents' views of themselves as disciplinarians (Table 5.9); at 11 and 21 years, how the mothers' rated their own health (feeling

Table 5.8. *Disciplinary methods used, 15 months, and 4 and 11 years, Down's syndrome and controls*

	15 months	4 years	11 years
Child smacked by mother	+	+	+
Child smacked by father			+
Sent to bed early		+	+
Sent out of the room		+	+
Given rewards			+
Closely supervised	+	+	+

Table 5.9. *Parents' views on discipline, 4 and 11 years, Down's syndrome and controls (percentages)*

	4 years	11 years
Parents agree about upbringing	+	+
Parents consistent on discipline		+
Father stricter		+
Mother stricter		+
Mother happy about her handling of children	+	+
Mother believes in smacking	+	
Mother believes smacking does good	+	
Little smacking for any child in family		+
Mother's permissiveness score	+	

Table 5.10. *Child factors, 15 months, and 4 and 11 years, Down's syndrome and controls (percentages)*

	15 months	4 years	11 years
Manageability		+	+
Gets into mischief		+	+
Has tantrums	+	+	
Amenability rating	+		
Personality rating			+

Table 5.11. *Outcome measures, 15 months, and 4 and 11 years, Down's syndrome and controls (percentages)*

	4 years	11 years	21 years
Cooperativeness			+
Manageability	+	+	+
Behaviour problems (many/few)			+

depressed/run down), since an ill or exhausted mother might have had greater difficulty in exercising discipline; and also a number of factors relating to the child (Table 5.10). These were related, as appropriate, to ratings made at 4, 11 and 21 years of their child's cooperativeness, manageability and number of behaviour problems (see Table 5.11). These ratings were individually related to cooperativeness and manageability at 11 and 21 years, and to frequency of behaviour problems at 21 years. Manageability, which was rated at 4, 11 and 21 years, was also correlated across ages. The expectation was that there would be a significant relationship between the disciplinary approaches used by the mothers and outcome in terms of cooperativeness, manageability, and presence or absence of behaviour problems in their children.

The first analyses concerned the relationships between child characteristics at one age and the dependent variables at later ages. The results are shown in Table 5.12. The controls tended to be easier to manage at age 11 if they had had few tantrums at 4, and the Down's syndrome young people were easier to manage if they had had few tantrums at 15 months. The Down's syndrome young people were found to be more cooperative at 21 years, if they had been easy to manage at 4 and if, at 11 years, they had kept out of mischief and been cooperative. Tantrums at 15 months showed the same trend, of greater cooperativeness where tantrums were fewer, but did not quite reach significance. The controls were seen as more cooperative at age 21 if they had had few tantrums at 4 and kept out of

Table 5.12. *Significant associations between disciplinary methods and child factors, Down's syndrome and controls*

| | Level of significance | |
	DS	Controls
Easier to manage at 11 years if		
At 4, rarely had tantrums	n.s.	[0.053][3]
Easier to manage at 21 years if		
At 15 months rarely had tantrums	0.019[1]	n.s.
More cooperative at 21 years if		
At 15 months, rarely had tantrums	[0.075][3]	n.s.
At 4 years, easy to manage	0.004[3]	[0.060}[1]
At 4 years, rarely had tantrums	n.s.	0.043[3]
At 11 years, kept out of mischief	0.043[3]	0.047[1]
At 11 years, was cooperative	0.048[2]	n.s.

1. Fisher's Exact Test.
2. McNemar's Test.
3. Continuity Adjusted χ^2.
Square brackets indicate associations which are almost significant at $P < 0.05$.

mischief at 11, whilst being easy to manage at 4, although not quite significant, showed the same trend.

Overall then, there was a tendency for those who were cooperative and easily managed, who kept out of mischief and were not subject to tantrums, to be more cooperative and easy to manage at later stages of their lives. Some consistency and regularity was shown in the behaviour of these young people.

Next to be considered were the relationships between the ratings of manageability and cooperativeness at 11 and 21 years, and of behaviour problems at age 21, with the earlier ratings of parents' usage of, and attitudes to, discipline. Only three significant results were obtained (see Table 5.13. The controls were easier to manage at age 11 if, at 4 years, the mother had believed in smacking, and more cooperative at age 21 if the mother had been the stricter parent. In the Down's syndrome group there were fewer behaviour problems at age 21 if, at 4 years, there had been little smacking for any child in the family. No other factor – smacking by mother or father, sending the child to bed early or out of the room, using rewards, whether the mother believed smacking did good or had confidence in her child-rearing methods, agreement between the parents on the child's upbringing, or the mother's health – could be shown to have any relationship with later behaviour.

Table 5.13. *Significant associations between disciplinary methods and manageability, cooperativeness and behaviour problems, Down's syndrome and controls*

	Level of significance	
	DS	Controls
11 years – easier to manage if At 4, mother believed in smacking	n.s.	0.044
21 years – more cooperative if At 11, mother the stricter parent	n.s.	0.034
21 years – fewer behaviour problems if At 4, little smacking in the home	0.050	n.s.

Table 5.14. *Discipline scales, 15 months, 4, 11 and 21 years*

	15 months	4 years	11 years	21 years
Ways of dealing with				
Sleep disturbance	+			
Destructiveness	+			
Tantrums	+	+		
Mischief		+	+	
Habits			+	+
Uses				
Smacking	+	+	+	
Other disciplinary methods		+	+	
Threats			+	+
Rewards			+	+

+ indicates items combined at each age to make the Discipline Scale. Thus, the Discipline Scale for 15 months consisted of the mothers' responses to questions on how they dealt with sleep disturbance, destructiveness, tantrums, and their use of smacking.

Since individual disciplinary methods had not been shown to affect behaviour, they were combined into Discipline Scales (see Table 5.14). Scores differed significantly between the Down's syndrome and control groups at 15 months, 4 and 11 years ($P < 0.01$) with in every case mothers of the Down's syndrome children being less strict than were those of the controls. At 21 years there was insufficient overlap between the groups to make a comparison meaningful. Scores on these scales for the Down's syndrome group were then related to cooperativeness, manageability and behaviour problems at age 21. None of the relationships was significant.

Table 5.15. *Associations between mother's attitude at 11 and 21 years, with mother's attitude at 11 and cooperation at 11 and 21, Downs syndrome and controls*

	M.att., 11	Coop 11	Coop 21
DS			
M.att., 11		$P = 0.005$	$P = 0.007$
M.att., 21	n.s.	n.s.	n.s.
Controls			
M.att., 11		n.s.	$P = 0.055$
M.att., 21	$P = 0.021$	n.s.	$P = 0.0013$

M.att., mother's attitude; coop, cooperation.

The failure to find evidence of systematic relationships between parental handling and later behaviour was unexpected and puzzling. In seeking an explanation, an earlier study by Caldwell (1964) seemed, perhaps, relevant. Caldwell studied, amongst other things, the methods of toilet training experienced by a group of young normal children and attempts to relate the use of these methods to the children's later psychological development. She is unable to demonstrate the connections that have been commonly held to exist between these factors (e.g., between a rigid toilet training regime and later obsessionality). The absence of such effects, Caldwell believes, must be due to other intervening factors, and she points to the potential importance of the 'inter-personal context' in which such training was carried out. It seems reasonable to suppose that something similar could be playing a part in the present case. Although, in the present study, the questionnaire was not designed with this in view there was one item, intended to bridge the transition from the inquiry about basic living skills to that of behaviour and management, which asked 'How would you describe N as a person now?'. This was an open-ended question, and the mothers' replies were recorded verbatim. Later, the replies were divided into three groups: those in which the mother had made only positive comments, those in which she had made both positive and negative comments, and those containing only negative comments. Because there were so few of the latter they were combined with the comments containing both positive and negative aspects, and this bipolar factor (labelled 'Mother's Attitude') at 11 and 21 years was related to measures of cooperation at each age. Results for both the Down's syndrome and control groups are given in Table 5.15.

In the Down's syndrome group, mother's attitude at 11 years was related to cooperativeness not only at 11 but also at 21 years. The mother's attitude at age 11 was not, however, related to her attitude at age 21; neither was her attitude at 21 related to cooperativeness at 21; nor was cooperativeness at 11 related to the mother's attitude at 21 (suggesting that it was not the child's cooperativeness at 11 years that resulted at 21 in a positive attitude in the mother). So, although not related to her attitude at age 21, mother's attitude at 11 years was related to cooperativeness in the young person at 21 years. In addition, while cooperativeness at 21 years was associated with cooperativeness at 11 years ($P = 0.048$), the association with mother's attitude at 11 years was the stronger one. Although the findings can be regarded only as tentative, they suggest that a positive attitude on the part of the mother of a child with Down's syndrome may have a role in facilitating his or her later cooperativeness.

In the controls the position was somewhat different. Mother's attitude at 11 years was not significantly related to cooperation at either 11 or 21 years but was significantly related to her attitude at 21 years, which in turn was related to cooperation at that time.

Discussion

Behaviours

While parents realise that Down's syndrome implies at least some degree of learning disability, many are reassured by friends and acquaintances, if not by professionals, with the idea that 'these children' are loveable, affectionate, good natured, friendly and so on. This stereotype has been challenged by Rollin (1946) and Blacketer-Simmonds (1953), who find people with Down's syndrome to be less docile and more mischievous than those with other forms of learning disability, but some other studies have found some truth in the early stereotype. In two very large studies, using data drawn from the 1966 census of institutionalised residents in the United States, people with Down's syndrome were rated significantly less often on maladaptive behaviour such as hyperactivity and aggression (Moore, Thuline & Capes 1968; Johnson & Abelson 1969). More recently, children with Down's syndrome are seen as more affectionate and outgoing than are children with other forms of learning disabilities (Gibbs & Thorpe 1983), and more positive in mood (although also less persistent and more distractible) than the standardisation sample of non-disabled children (Gunn & Cuskelly 1991). Gibson (1978) in a thorough and wide ranging examination of personality in Down's syndrome individuals, concludes that 'behavioural difficulties in younger Down's syndome samples is less common and less acute than for other young moderately to seriously mentally retarded', though he feels that this may change with adulthood.

In the present study, most parents described their young and adult children in positive terms as affectionate, loveable, kind and friendly, the figures being very similar to those for the controls. In the Down's syndrome group, stubbornness was also a common description at both ages. The minority seen as difficult and troublesome was always smaller in the Down's syndrome group, though the differences were not significant. Mothers in the two groups may have approached the questions about behavioural problems from a somewhat different stand point, but it is salutary to remember that difficulties in families can also occur in the absence of disability.

Most in the Down's syndrome group were said, at each age, to be cooperative and manageable and this proportion increased over time, so that by age 21 the mothers were finding the management of their son or daughter an easier task than it had been in the past. This finding, supported also by that of Holmes (1988), that the Down's syndrome young people became easier to manage as they became older, contrasts with the suggestion by Gibson (1978, p. 138) that the Down's syndrome person is at his or her best in the middle years of childhood and shows 'markedly less attractive behaviours' as he or she grows older. That this was not the case in the present sample, and that their parents found that, on the contrary, their young people were easier to handle as they matured, was a welcome development. Difficulties of management certainly existed, and these tended to be concentrated in the more disabled of the group (although there were many others in the more disabled range who were not particularly difficult). Nevertheless, those with higher ability (IQ 35+), although they might need tactful handling from time to time, did not present their parents with serious problems of management.

In both groups of children, habits were common and in the Down's syndrome group many of these persisted into adulthood, only the most able being exempted. On the whole, however, these habits were the less severe and distressing ones, such as nail biting in childhood, and masturbation and rocking at both ages. Self-injury, although not unknown in people with Down's syndrome, was relatively rare and where it did occur was usually minor in degree.

Most of the particular behaviour problems asked about, and reported on, were minor or infrequent, affecting around one-third of the children and young people. The exception to this was rebelliousness, affecting half to two-thirds, supporting the often stated view that for all their good humour and pleasantness Down's syndrome people are characterised by stubbornness. Efforts to link stubbornness with disciplinary methods – the use of a variety of punishments and rewards – yielded nothing except for a non-significant trend towards more rebelliousness in those who had been smacked more frequently. While these figures are far from conclusive they at least do not lend support to any idea that rebelliousness may be dealt with by firm, physical punishment.

Discipline

Parents deal with their children – loving and encouraging, checking and disciplining – in ways which they hope will help the children to be, and to grow up to be, pleasant and positive people, and to make for harmonious family life. For any parent this is a hazardous undertaking, fraught with imponderables; where the child has a disability the outlook is even more uncertain. Parents of a disabled child have fewer examples to look to, fewer friends, neighbours or relatives with a comparable child to watch and compare notes with, and fewer readily available sources of advice to call on. One mother of a Down's syndrome girl, commenting at 4 years on how little advice she had received, said 'I didn't know what to do, nobody told me anything, I just had to fish around by myself. As it's turned out she's quite good, but I might have done her harm'.

With few known facts on which to base advice about the most profitable ways of managing a child with Down's syndrome, a longitudinal study, such as the present one, offers the opportunity to look at the disciplinary methods the parents used, to compare these with later outcomes, and to examine whether some methods were associated with better outcomes than others. In the event, the study provides very little in the way of guide lines. No one way of handling the children and young people, neither punishment nor any variety of punishment, nor the use of rewards, has been shown to be clearly better than any other. However, some, although not invariable, relationships were found between ratings of the children at different ages, showing that those rated as easy, pleasant people at one age were likely to be rated similarly at another. Some consistency then was shown between behaviours at different ages; the parents' efforts to influence behaviours could not be shown to have had much effect at all.

These results cut across common beliefs. Parents expect that they will be able to influence their children's behaviour: that praise or reward will result in the child becoming more 'good'; more commonly, that punishment will result in the child becoming less 'bad'. 'All parents have in common that they intend to be effective in whatever means they use to instil "goodness" in their children' (Newson & Newson, 1989, p. 21). Professionals, too, have similar expectations and are prepared, when they see parental methods failing, to advise the parents to adopt others, possibly more subtle, but still based on principles very similar to those underpinning the methods adopted by the parents. Both groups expect to be able to channel the child towards behaviours that are seen as both positive for him or herself, and acceptable to society at large. This states the case simplistically, and parents and professionals recognise that other factors will have a bearing on what the child does and how he or she behaves at any one time. Nevertheless, broadly they believe that their efforts will make a significant contribution to the enhancement of the child's social and moral development.

Before attempting to explain the present findings, which appear to support few of the expectations described above, it is necessary to register some caution regarding the status of the present study and the data derived from it. Firstly, the numbers in the study are very small, which restricts the scope of statistical analyses that can be applied. If numbers had been larger it may have been possible to do more fine-grained analyses – e.g., to look at the effectiveness of specific forms of punishment or reward, more particularly to look at the interaction of effects, which might have resulted in richer and more informative data than it has been possible to provide here. Secondly, the research instrument used (the questionnaire schedule) may not have been sufficiently sensitive to allow differences in parental approaches to emerge. Thirdly, since all the data are derived from the mothers' reports – due to resource constraints on the 21 year study no other agency (e.g., the young people's day centres) was approached – any continuities seen could be construed as continuities of the mothers' perceptions, and not necessarily of their offsprings' behaviour. Finally, there may yet be further analyses of the data to be done that would yield positive results, although it is believed that the major ones have already been carried out.

That having been said, it still remains that, within its limits, the present study has provided data that point to the conclusion that the major predictors of behaviour, and of ease of management, in these adults with Down's syndrome were similar traits seen in earlier childhood, and that these were little affected by the disciplinary methods that the parents used. The question then arises as to whether this is an isolated finding, and how far it accords with those from other studies.

Since longitudinal studies in the area of learning difficulties are thin on the ground, studies of non-disabled children will be discussed first; in particular, two major studies – those carried out in New York (Thomas & Chess 1977; Chess & Thomas 1984) and in Nottingham (Newson & Newson 1963, 1968, 1989). Both are longitudinal studies, from infancy to adulthood, and are based on substantial populations (133 and more than 700 respectively). Both have included the exploration of the relationships to be seen between parental practices and later child temperament and behaviour. The studies differ from each other not only geographically but also in the social class background of their populations: in the New York study the families were almost exclusively professional and predominantly Jewish, and the children's mean IQs were over 120 (Chess & Thomas 1984, p. 51); the Nottingham sample was composed of families from a spread of social class that was reasonably representative of the area, and the children's IQs represented a wide range with a mean of just under 100 (Newson & Newson 1977).

In the New York study, using a variety of measures and of statistical approaches, some temperamental continuities, from childhood to adulthood, emerged. Temperament scores (difficult-easy) at three years were significantly related to adult temperament scores, even when three-year adjustment and parent attitude scores were controlled for, and were related also to adult adjustment. 'Adjustment' at 3 was almost invariably related to adult adjustment. However, 'maternal attitudes' at 3 years were even more highly related to adult adjustment. 'Maternal attitudes' consisted of a set of eight cluster variables including strictness, inter-parental conflict and standards of living, of which inter-parental conflict emerged as especially important. The authors conclude: 'Outstanding in the high risk factors in childhood for a relatively poor overall adjustment in early adult life were difficult temperament, parental conflict, the presence of a behaviour disorder and the global adjustment score at three years (Chess & Thomas 1984, p. 99).

In this study then, measurements of temperament and adjustment in childhood were good predictors of the same factors in adult life, and the data from the present study are in agreement with this conclusion. In addition, however, is the finding of the effect of parental attitudes and practices, although the major influence here seems to lie more with the parents' relationship with each other than with parental disciplinary approaches to their children (although the children's *response* to disciplinary measures, a factor labelled 'discipline', also featured in some of the analyses).

In the Nottingham study, children who were rated as difficult at 11 years were more likely to be described as troublesome at 16, and more likely to go on to acquire a criminal record (both significant at $P < 0.001$), than were those not difficult at age 11 (Newson & Newson 1989). Here again, there is some consistency in at least one kind of behaviour from one age to another. The more interesting of the Newsons' findings, however, relate to those concerned with the relationship between early parental disciplinary methods and later behaviour. Children who at 11 years were physically punished on a regular basis (once a week or more), where one parent at least used an instrument to punish, and especially where these two factors were combined with the mother's reliance on corporal punishment, were more likely to be seen as troublesome at age 16 and more likely eventually to acquire a criminal record than were children not subjected to these regimes. This association held even where sex, family size and social class were controlled for. The extent to which parents were prepared to deceive the child (including the use of idle threats in order to exert discipline), a factor the Newsons entitled 'bamboozlement', was also associated with poorer outcomes. The Newsons are careful not to draw the conclusion that punishment and deception *cause* troublesomeness and delinquency in the children, but they point to the fallacy of the dictum. 'Spare the rod and spoil the child'; their data do not show smacking and beating to be effective ways to teach children to behave better.

In the Nottingham study, then, there are some clear associations between the type of discipline exerted by the parents and later behavioural outcome, even if this was not the outcome expected or intended by the parents.

In the present Down's syndrome study in Surrey, the criterion of smacking used by Newson & Newson (1989) (distinguishing children who were smacked once a week or more from those who were smacked less) was considered. In the control group, 13% were smacked once a week or more at 11 years, compared with 18% in Nottingham, but no relationship could be seen with how cooperative or easy to manage they were at 21. In the Down's syndrome group, 21% were smacked once a week or more at 11 years; at age 21, all the relationships – with uncooperativeness, being difficult to manage or rebellious, and having two or more behaviour problems – showed, as in Nottingham, more problems in those smacked more frequently, but the figures do not reach significance.

Besides these two studies of non-disabled children, there are two longitudinal studies of children with learning disabilities that present data relevant to the present inquiry. The first is that of Richardson and his colleagues (Richardson, Koller & Katz, 1985), of children with mild learning difficulties in Scotland; the second that of Cunningham, Sloper, Byrne and associates (Byrne *et al.* 1988) of children with Down's syndrome in Manchester. Richardson *et al.* (1985) report on a population sample of children with mild learning difficulties, studied during childhood and followed up at 16 and 22 years. Each child with mild learning difficulties was individually matched for age, sex, area of residence and social class with a child without learning difficulties. Behaviour disturbance in the child, and the stability of his or her upbringing were each rated on five-point scales. There was significantly more behaviour disturbance in the children with mild learning difficulties than in the comparison group, and in both groups behaviour disturbance increased as stability of upbringing decreased. When stability of upbringing was controlled for there was no significant difference in behaviour disturbance between the groups, nor did the presence of central nervous system involvement in the learning difficulties group contribute towards behaviour disturbance. Finally, the authors conclude that the greater degree of instability in the families of the children with mild learning difficulties was not due to the presence of these children, but was more likely to result from other factors, such as low income, large family and 'various forms of social pathology' (Richardson *et al.* 1985, p. 7). Thus, from this study, the main conclusion is that the behavioural disturbance exhibited by this group of young people is probably not due to their intellectual disability but to the stressful conditions they experienced as they grew up.

The Manchester Down's syndrome study (Byrne *et al.* 1988) has direct lines of comparison with the present one in Surrey, and has the advantage of larger numbers (although the children reported on were younger, not yet having reached adolescence). Again, some consistency of behaviour over time was noted: 75% of mothers who had been concerned about their Down's syndrome child's behaviour at ages ranging from 2 to 10 years were still concerned about behaviour two to three years later. Factors which were related to behavioural problems included unemployment in the father, a poor relationship between mother and child, and low developmental status of the child. Despite one of the avowed aims of the study being to examine the factors that affected later development, efforts to relate disciplinary methods to later outcome were largely unproductive; the only associations found were of less problem behaviour where the mother had felt happy about how she handled the child ($r = 0.23$, $P < 0.005$) and more problems where she had threatened to send the child away ($r = 0.22$, $P < 0.05$, P. Sloper, personal communication). Once again, child behaviour showed some uniformity from one age to another, and the disciplinary methods exerted by the mother were not shown to have had a pronounced effect on the future behaviour of the child.

Overall these studies show that in all the groups of children considered, whether disabled or non-disabled, some, although by no means invariable, behavioural consistency is seen across ages; family conflict or disturbance is associated with later disturbance or poor adjustment in the children; and physical punishment, which is intended to make the child see the error of his ways and behave better, has not been shown to do so.

With the exception of family disturbance (which did not occur in sufficient numbers to be a significant factor in the present study) the findings in the Surrey study, so far as they go, are in accordance with those from the other studies. Given the limitations of the present study, we are not in a position yet to offer detailed advice to families on how they should handle their children with Down's syndrome. But we can suggest that, as for non-disabled children, a harmonious, loving family is likely to give the children a good start in life; and, however tempting it may seem in the short term, physical punishment is unlikely to make naughty children grow up into pleasant well-adjusted adults.

SIX

Focusing on the individual

In previous chapters, we have looked at the achievements of the Down's syndrome group, their abilities and accomplishments, and at their behaviour. Here, we look at their own lives as children and as adults, at home and out of the home. Current philosophy envisages people with learning disabilities living in the community and functioning, as far as possible, as ordinary members of the community; we wanted to see how far these aims had been achieved, what the difficulties were in achieving them, and what were the views of those concerned with the group about what should be done to help them.

Health can affect all other areas of a person's life, and we began by asking how the health of the children and young people had been during the intervals between 4 and 11 years, and between 11 and 21 years (see Table 6.1).

Health

Most in both the Down's syndrome and control groups, and at age 11 and 21, were seen as having good health, a finding similar to that in other studies (Holmes 1988; Shepperdson 1992). At age 21 one-quarter in each group (Down's syndrome 29%; controls 27%) were said to be very healthy. More of the children in the Down's syndrome group had poor health but the difference from the controls is not significant. By 21 years two of these delicate children (both girls) had died. Two profoundly disabled young men were at 21 years again said to be delicate, as was also another in this group who had not been seen at 11 years. A further young man, severely but not profoundly disabled, was in poor health at 11 and at 21 years and died soon after the 21 year interview. However, seven of the 11 who had been seen as delicate as children were considered at age 21 to be quite robust.

As children, just under one-third in each group had suffered a serious illness. Some in both groups had had the childhood ailments such as measles, mumps, chickenpox and scarlet fever; one in each group had had gastroenteritis, three Down's syndrome and one control child had had bronchitis (one mother in the Down's syndrome group said 'She's been in

Table 6.1. *Health since last seen, age 11 and 21, Down's syndrome and controls (percentages)*

	11 years		21 years	
	DS	Control	DS	Control
Good	74	94	88	94
Poor	26	6	12	6
Had serious illness	30	27	N.A.	N.A.
Had serious accident	9	33**	N.A.	N.A.

See Table 2.1 for definitions, and Table 3.4 for significance levels.

hospital for it so often I've lost count'), one Down's syndrome child suffered from an enlarged kidney and another had had a bowel obstruction that had kept him in hospital for nine months. One child with Down's syndrome and three controls had had surgery for appendicitis, one control for adenoids. Four children with Down's syndrome had had pneumonia (one of them four times) and three had been hospitalised for heart problems; neither of these ailments had been suffered by the controls. One control child had had meningitis twice, and another was diabetic. The severity of the illnesses, therefore, seemed to have been rather more pronounced in the Down's syndrome group, but the number of children who had suffered serious illnesses was comparable between the two groups.

However, significantly more of the control children had suffered a serious accident: four had had cuts requiring stitching, three had broken arms and one a nose, one had fallen and been concussed, one had been scalded, one sustained an eye injury, one girl had had a needle in her elbow, and another was involved in a road traffic accident. In the Down's syndrome group, three children had had falls, one from a pony, resulting in concussion; one had been in a road traffic accident. Probably this difference is due to the greater freedom and adventurousness of the controls: almost all of the controls but only four of the Down's syndrome children could ride a bicycle, and all of the controls were allowed out of their garden to go into the neighbourhood or further, compared with only one-third of the children with Down's syndrome.

At age 21, a quarter in each group were subject to colds and flu; about half got these only occasionally but the young people with Down's syndrome got coughs rather more often than did the controls, and five, compared with none of the controls, were subject to bronchitis (see Table 6.2). Heart ailments too were much more frequent in the Down's syndrome group, affecting 15 young people (37%, similar to the 32% in Buckley & Sacks' (1987) teenage sample and 40% in Rowe & Uchida's (1961) study,

Table 6.2. *Minor illnesses in last year, age 11 and 21, Down's syndrome and controls (percentages)*

	Colds/Flu		Coughs		Bronchitis	
	DS	Control	DS	Control	DS	Control
< 1 p.a.	24	30	42	60	88	100
1 – 2 p.a.	49	43	44	33	7	0
> 2 p.a.	27	27	14	7	5	0

p.a., per annum.

citation from Gibson 1978) compared with none of the controls. Four young men had serious heart conditions (one dying soon after the interview) and five young women and one young man had more minor conditions. Five young people, three men and two women, had had heart conditions in the past but these were not thought to affect now: most had had minor heart conditions in the past which were no longer troublesome, but one young woman had undergone successful heart surgery. Three young men with Down's syndrome (but no controls) had epilepsy, which had begun at 10, 12 and 14 years. Two of these were in the profoundly, and one in the severely, disabled group; in two cases the young men were in care and the epileptic fits were controlled by medication, but the young man living at home had fits about once or twice a fortnight despite medication and very careful medical supervision. Apart from this, seven Down's syndrome young people and three controls were on some form of regular medication – the contraceptive pill (one Down's syndrome and two control young women), sleeping, iron or thyroid tablets, tranquillisers, a low dose antibiotic for acne ('we have queried this but they say it's quite safe, and as soon as we stop it it comes back'), each taken by one Down's syndrome person, while another young woman with Down's syndrome was on Largactyl and anti-depressants.

Over half in each group were affected by other medical problems: in the Down's syndrome group nearly a third (29%) had skin problems – acne, boils, dry skin or, in three cases, dry scalp, athlete's foot, and a weeping navel. One young man was diabetic, another had a thyroid condition, two had trouble with their teeth, and one of them, an epileptic young man, had gingivitis; one profoundly disabled young woman caused a lump on her tongue by repeated biting and this was removed; and one young man had polycythaemia. Two of the profoundly disabled young men had had pneumonia; one of these had also had urinary infections, problems with his teeth and had had a tumour removed from his buttock. The other (of whom it was said when he was 6 weeks old, 'Down's syndrome is the least of his

Table 6.3. *Days' illness and visits to doctors in last year, age 21,
Down's syndrome (percentages)*

Number	Days' illness		Visits to GP		OP appointment	
	DS	Control	DS	Control	DS	Control
None	72	39	33	36	53	56
1 – 3	8	29	42	39	38	30
4 – 6	15	18	18	18	7	7
7 – 10	5	3	5	0	2	7
12	0	0	2	7	0	0
21 – 28	0	11	0	0	0	0

OP, out-patient.

worries') was almost a medical textbook in himself: having had pneumonia
twice, salmonella infections twice, chest infections three times, chickenpox,
shingles and measles, consolidation of the lung, was Australian-antigen
positive and, as a consequence of his pica, had had a rectal obstruction
requiring surgical intervention at which pieces of fibre, plastic and string
were removed. By contrast, four of the controls had mild skin problems,
two had sustained broken legs, one concussion, two had hayfever and one
asthma, one an in-growing toenail and three had had cystitis, thrush and
an infection of the Fallopian tube.

Despite these more serious medical problems, the young people with
Down's syndrome had had fewer days' illness in the past year than had
the controls, and they had had no more appointments with their own or
with hospital doctors than the controls (see Table 6.3). Contrary to Murdoch's (1985) finding, that children with Down's syndrome with congenital
heart disease show no greater morbidity, including contact with GPs
(general practioners), than those without heart conditions, the majority of
GP and hospital out-patient contacts in the present group were made by
those with some current degree of heart problem. Those with problems
saw their GP on average 3.6 times over the past year, compared with 1.9
for those without heart problems, and the figures for hospital appointments
were 2.9 and 0.7, respectively. Nearly half of the children in each group
had been admitted to hospital at least once in the previous seven years (see
Table 6.4). Only one child (the girl with Down's syndrome who had had
numerous admissions for bronchitis) had been in hospital more than three
times, and overall there was little difference between the groups in the frequency of admissions.

However, where the adults were concerned, and in contrast with the
figures for out-patient appointments, the young people with Down's syndrome had been admitted to hospital rather more often, three, compared

Table 6.4. *Hospital admissions, 4–11 and 11–21, Down's syndrome and controls (percentages)*

	11 years		21 years	
	DS	Control	DS	Control
None	57	52	55	54
One	29	35	25	40
Two	2	8	13	3
Three or more	12	5	7	3

Table 6.5. *Weight problems, age 21, Down's syndrome and controls, (percentages)*

	DS	Control
None	52	63
Slightly overweight	22	20
Definitely overweight	22	10
Slightly underweight	2	7
Definitely underweight	2	0

with none of the controls, having been admitted twice or more in the last year, and eight (20%), compared with only two controls, twice or more in the last ten years. Nevertheless, apart from three young men with Down's syndrome who had each spent around 14 weeks altogether in hospital (two were the profoundly disabled young men referred to above, and another, one who had been in a road traffic accident), there was little difference between the groups in the length of their hospital stay.

Besides inquiring about illnesses and hospitals we asked about weight, and about hearing and vision (see Table 6.5). Just over half the young people with Down's syndrome and nearly two-thirds of the controls were said to be of normal weight. Forty-four per cent of the young people with Down's syndrome were thought to be overweight, a figure that coincides with that given by Buckley & Sacks (1987) (although in Holmes' study (1988) 66% of the rather older adults were said to be overweight). In the Down's syndrome group, six men and 12 women (27% and 63%, respectively) were said to be overweight, compared with four men and five women (31% and 29%) in the controls. The difference between the sexes in the Down's syndrome young people was significant at $P<0.01$, and that between the Down's syndrome and control groups was significant $(P<0.05)$

Table 6.6. *Vision and hearing, age 21, Down's syndrome (percentages)*

	Vision		Hearing	
	DS	Control	DS	Control
None	29	83	86	100
Wears spectacles/aid (or should)	64	17	7	0
Very poor	7	0	7	0

between the women but not between the men; nor was the difference between the combined sexes of the two groups significant.

Nearly three-quarters of the young people with Down's syndrome, compared with one-sixth of the controls, had difficulties with vision (see Table 6.6). Nearly half (42%) wore spectacles and just over a fifth (22%) should have done so but refused to wear them, comparable figures for the controls being 7% and 10%, respectively. The figures for poor vision in the Down's syndrome group are rather higher than those in the Buckley & Sacks' (1987) study, where 48% of the under 14s and 59% of the 14 to 17 age group had poor vision. This suggests that poor vision, or the detection of it, increases with increasing age but this is not supported by data from Holmes' (1988) study, where mean age was 28 years and poor vision was reported in only 29%. In the present study, less than a fifth of the young people with Down's syndrome (but none of the controls) had hearing problems: two had poor hearing, one young woman wore a hearing aid and another should have done so but refused. This relatively low level of reported hearing loss is perhaps surprising, since much higher levels have been reported in Down's syndrome people – e.g., Nolan *et al.* (1980) reports 69% of the Down's syndrome people they studied as having a hearing loss. Just over two-thirds of the group, in the present study, had had their hearing tested and it may be that hearing defects had been missed in at least some, such as the three profoundly disabled people in the untested group. However, even if (as, from personal contact, seems unlikely) all this untested group in fact had hearing problems this would give an overall rate in the cohort of less than half (44%). Holmes (1988) finds only 10% of her group reported as having hearing problems, and it may be that this level is likely to be reported in the kind of inquiry discussed both here and by Holmes, where the information is derived from reports by relatives or carers and not from the results of hearing tests.

None of the health factors – illnesses, hospital visits, hearing, vision or weight problems – could be seen to have adversely affected the young person's intellectual progress. The only association between health and ability was found for those young people described as delicate, where all the mean ability scores (IQ, language, reading and arithmetic) were well below that expected. Very poor general health did seem to be to some extent associated with greater intellectual difficulty, although the association did not hold up in multivariate analyses (see Chapter 3).

Overall the differences in health between the Down's syndrome and control groups were not as striking as had been expected. This applied not only to subjective estimates, such as those for weight, and for general health, which as we suggested (Carr 1975) may be explained in part by parents' expectations of more serious problems. Such an explanation is less able to account for the similarities in the number who had other medical problems, or were taking medicines, or the number of times that young people saw their own doctor or had a hospital appointment. The findings are in general agreement with those from Buckley & Sacks (1987) and from Shepperdson's (1984) study, which show most teenagers with Down's syndrome to have reasonably good health. The 10% of adults with delicate health in Holmes (1988) study is also similar to the 12% found here, and it seems that most families do not see their Down's syndrome offspring as markedly unhealthy. A small number (three in the present study) certainly suffered very serious health problems, but apart from these, health in the remainder of the group was little different from that of their non-disabled peers.

Staying at home and going out

As children leave their babyhood behind all parents face a conflict between the need to provide, on the one hand, adequate protection and, on the other, sufficient freedom so that the children can move towards independence. This dilemma is enhanced when the child has a disability, and parents are even more uncertain as to how able he or she is to take responsibility; it is common for parents of disabled children to be described as over-restrictive. Nevertheless, parents do allow their disabled children more freedom, and the children do become more independent, as they get older (see Table 6.7).

Whereas at 4 years less than half the children with Down's syndrome (44%) could be left to play on their own, in a room with the mother nearby, for as long as half an hour, by 11 years over half the children (57%), and by 21 four-fifths (82%) could be left alone in the house for at least a few minutes while the mother popped out. Just under half the 11 year olds would never be left for a minute, and this remained true at age 21 for just under a fifth. Even higher figures are given from the Hampshire and Welsh researches: of the children, 80% (Hampshire) and 62% (Welsh), and of the older teenagers (14–17 years) and young adults, 32% and 31%,

Table 6.7. *Able to cope in and out of home, 11 and 21 years, Down's syndrome (percentages)*

	11 years	21 years
At home alone		
Never	43	18
A minute or two	40	15
Half to one hour	17	41
Half day to all day	0	26
Out of house alone		
Never	14	10
In garden only	48	46
Neighbourhood	33	24
To nearby places	5	15
Further	0	4

respectively, were never left (Buckley & Sacks 1987; Shepperdson 1992). In the Surrey group at each age, while those 'never left' contained all the most severely disabled they also included some who were more able: amongst the children, five girls and two boys with IQs in the top one-third for the group (IQ 40+); amongst the adults, two capable young people, one young woman whose (ill) mother said she would be too worried herself to leave her daughter, and one charming, but slightly scatty, young man whose mother said she could leave him for ten minutes at the most. Three parents were particularly worried about leaving their young people for fear of what would happen if someone came to the door.

> We tell her to put the chain on and not to answer the door. *She's* safe enough, it's other people we worry about.

> If we're out in the garden we lock the front door. We're frightened what would happen if someone came to the door, she'd go off with anybody.

More than a third of the children were able to go beyond the garden, most just around the local neighbourhood but two competent girls could go further afield. Most of this group of 16 children allowed beyond the garden were of above average ability but three, with more limited ability, lived in quiet areas with a corner shop nearby that they could go to on their own. One mother had considerable confidence in allowing her child to go out despite the possible problems.

> He goes out with the dog sometimes and the dog won't let anyone near him, so if he's lost it's difficult for him to be brought home. He's not really allowed out of the fields around the house and he sticks with that pretty well.

Another, however, had had some alarming experiences.

> I did start letting him out to play football at one time and next thing I knew
> he was in [*nearby town*] and the police picked him up. The other kids came
> in and told me he'd gone off on his tricycle. Another time he let himself out
> of the house while I was there and disappeared; when I eventually found
> him he had crossed the main road and gone to a friend's house.

Ten years later over half the young people still could not be allowed
beyond the garden alone, and some had provided good reason why such
restrictions should be imposed. The young man described below was a five
day boarder at a large hospital and travelled daily to the day centre.

> One day when the group were going to catch the coach he must have
> got away from them and didn't get on the coach, and he walked to the
> day centre all by himself. They rang up from there and said 'We won't
> be responsible if he doesn't come with a proper escort' – we had no
> idea he wasn't on the coach and we were scared stiff. [*This is the same
> young man who as an 11 year old was concerned in the escapade on his
> tricycle to the nearby town.*]

Another young man was also confined to the garden, as far as this was
possible.

> He goes on walk-about sometimes, often to the next house. Twice he's
> got away from his centre; once he got on a bus and went to [*large
> nearby town*] and was found playing on the lifts, and once he was on a
> bus to [*another town*] and the conductor took him into the town and to
> the police station. Once, when he was at school, he got on the train to
> Waterloo and was stopped then because he hadn't got a ticket, and the
> police were called – they were very good.

One-fifth of the young people, all very capable, could make trips out of
their local neighbourhood, two of these, one young man and one young
woman, travelling considerable distances and coping with tickets and with
changes of buses and trains. Seventeen (41%) of the young people were
able to cross at least some roads although only six of these (15%) were
thought able to cross any road they encountered. All these six young people
had ability levels above the average (IQ 42+) but 12 others of similar levels
were not thought able to cross roads.

Clearly a number of factors besides the young person's ability are
involved in parents' decisions as to whether or not to allow more independence to their disabled offspring. Even the most able in this group were
not of normal ability, so factors which to mothers of normal children seem
manageable could become daunting barriers. One of these factors concerned the type of neighbourhood in which the person lived: those who
would not be allowed beyond the garden in an urban area might well be

allowed to roam further if they lived in the comparative safety of the countryside, particularly if they were well known in the area by local people who could be relied on to give help if it was needed. Another factor may have been the mother's own make-up, and how far her personality allowed her to let the young person take risks. We have no evidence on this point and are disinclined lightly to label mothers as 'overprotective' but in a few cases it certainly appeared as if the main thing restricting the young person's freedom was the mother's own fearfulness.

Interests and activities

At age 11 we asked whether the children had any special interests that occupied much of their spare time; at age 21, following the format used by Holmes (1988), we asked about a range of leisure activities the young people could have engaged in – a variety of sports, indoor occupations, household chores and cookery, outings, memberships of clubs and going to entertainments. We asked how frequently the young people did these things, from once a year or less to daily (see Table 6.8). Detailed questions on these topics were not asked at either age for the controls.

Table 6.8. *Interests and activities, 11 and 21, Down's syndrome and controls (percentages)*

	11 years		21 years	
	DS	Controls	DS	Controls
Sport				
One or more	14	68	80 (61)	81
Two or more	N.A.	N.A.	61 (37)	65
Indoor occupations				
Drawing ⎫	14	⎫ 40	68 (49)	N.A.
Books ⎭		⎭	85 (78)	N.A.
Board/table games	21	21	76 (39)	N.A.
Dolls/soldiers/cars	14	5	0	N.A.
TV	N.A.	N.A.	93 (90)	N.A.
Music	9	11	95 (93)	N.A.
Does household chores	N.A.	N.A.	93 (93)	92 (61)
Cooks				
Simple things	N.A.	N.A.	63 (54)	N.A.
More complex	N.A.	N.A.	2 (2)	81

(Main percentages in Table 6.8 and 6.9 indicate those ever involved: percentages in brackets, those involved once a week or more).

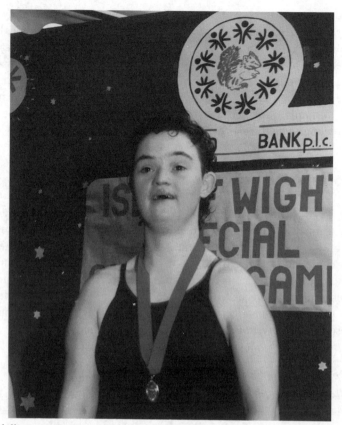

Medallist

At age 11, although sport was a major interest for the controls it was of little importance for those with Down's syndrome, apart from 9% who especially enjoyed swimming and 7% horse-riding. By 21 years four-fifths participated in some sport, three-fifths doing so at least once a week. Swimming was the most popular, engaged in by over half (58%) of the 21 year olds, with one-third swimming weekly or more often. One young woman regularly competed in international swimming events for the disabled, and had won numerous trophies, including a silver medal in the Special Olympics held in the United States, and was frequently featured in her local newspaper following these triumphs. Three had had to stop going to swimming baths because the chlorine affected their ears, breathing or skin, and it had been a blow to have to give up something they had enjoyed so much. More than a third enjoyed table tennis and organised games such as football, cricket and tennis. These figures are higher than those given by Holmes

(1988); it may be that this is due to the age difference between the two groups, and that people with Down's syndrome engage in fewer sporting activities as they get older – as indeed do those who are not disabled, in whom participation in both in- and out-door sport declines with age (Sports Council 1988). Those who did not take part in sport consisted, on the one hand, of four profoundly disabled young people and, on the other, of four who were relatively able and independent, who may have decided for themselves that sport was not for them.

Where indoor occupations were concerned, drawing, reading and handicrafts predominated for the 11 year old controls, while for the children with Down's syndrome, table top games – jigsaws, lego and dominoes – were in first place, enjoyed by just under a fifth, followed by drawing and reading, and by dolls and soldiers, each mentioned as an interest of six children. Perhaps surprisingly, music was mentioned as an interest for only three of the children with Down's syndrome. Many controls were said to have idiosyncratic interests (those not shared by a sufficient number to include in the table) – gardening, chess, music, dancing, babies (one boy and one girl), Scouts and Brownies, model making and electricity. In the Down's syndrome group the range of interests was much more restricted, although one boy, in the non-home-reared group, had an occupation not mentioned by any other mother in either group.

> Marbles. Its gone on for years and years. He makes them into whatever he wants and then he moves them around, for hours on end. They'll be soldiers and he'll march them up and down, or school children in class. The latest thing was Princess Anne's wedding, one marble was the bride and another the groom and the rest were bridesmaids and the congregation.

The more limited range of interests shown by the children with Down's syndrome, and the fact that over one-third (35%) compared with only 8% of the controls, were said to have no real interest the mother could identify, might be interpreted in terms of the Down's syndrome children's limited ability and developmental level. Apart from one boy said to love cars, no child with an IQ less than 30 was said to have any interest, but the remainder of this 'interest-less' group, three boys and three girls, had IQs of up to 55. So a low ability level seems to make it unlikely a child will engage in activities for their own sake, but higher levels of ability do not make it certain that they will – as is also seen in the controls, albeit a small number of them.

Indoor interests were not asked about for the adult controls but watching TV and listening to music were part of the daily routine for almost all the 21 year olds with Down's syndrome. These figures are very similar to those in Holmes' (1988) and in Buckley & Sacks' (1987) studies, as are also those for playing table games and drawing, though rather more of Holmes'

(older) and rather fewer of Buckley & Sacks' (younger) groups were interested in books. Putnam, Pueschel & Holman (1988) give lower figures,
apart from those for watching TV and listening to music: e.g. for those
participating weekly or more in sport 41%, and going to clubs 31%, and
to parties or dances 6%. Over 90% in both the Surrey and London studies
did household chores (only three very profoundly disabled, hospitalised
young people in the present study being excepted), three-quarters doing
these daily, whereas over a third of the controls did chores only with reluctance ('Not if he can help it'). Over half of the young people with Down's
syndrome could do simple cookery such as making a cup of tea or coffee,
or making toast or a sandwich but only one could do more than this – a
very competent young woman who could produce a creditable chilli con
carne or shepherds pie. Four-fifths of the controls were able to produce
cooked meals, at least for themselves, but five were non-proficient cooks,
one young woman being described by her mother as 'the only person I
know who has managed to burn a jelly'.

Outings

Nearly all the children in both groups were taken on outings (see Table
6.9) to films, theatres, museums, and picnics. Seven (20%) of the children

Table 6.9. *Outings, age 11, Down's syndrome and controls; age 21,*
Down's syndrome (percentages)

	11 years		21 years	
	DS	Control	DS	Control
Taken out to				
Films, theatre	69	57 ⎤		
Museums	71	38 ⎥ Outings	90 (27)	N.A.
Picnics	80	76 ⎥		
Swimming	60	57 ⎦		
Goes out				
Shopping				
Accompanied			93 (66)	N.A.
Alone			37 (32)	N.A.
To youth clubs				
Special			63 (49)	N.A.
Community			12 (10)	39 (0)
To dances				
Special			66 (32)	
Community			27 (10)	75 (11)

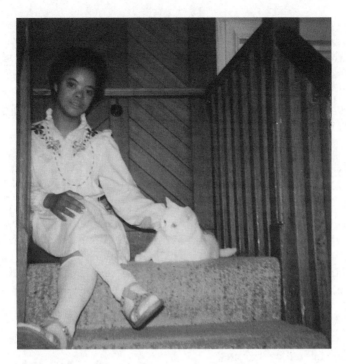

Disco dancer sitting out

with Down's syndrome and 10 (27%) of the controls only went out on picnics, while two in each group were not taken on any outings. As adults, almost all the young people went shopping when there was somebody to go with them, the two exceptions being one profoundly disabled young man living in a large hospital and one very independent young woman living away from home who shopped on her own and did not need an escort. Over a third were able to shop on their own, most of them quite often; these were young people with above average ability levels apart from one severely disabled young man (who died shortly after the interview) whose weekly outing was to the corner shop to fetch the Sunday papers. There were, however, nearly as many young people, again with similar ability levels, who did not shop alone, and clearly many other factors affect this, not only parental attitudes and anxieties but also the neighbourhood they live in, the proximity of the shops and the hazardousness of roads that have to be negotiated.

Almost two-thirds of the young people with Down's syndrome, like those in Holmes' (1988) study, went to leisure clubs in the evening and to their dances, while nearly a third went to dances in the community, many of them accompanying their parents who particularly enjoyed this type of activity and made sure the young people could enjoy them too. These young people were not necessarily the most able but included some whose parents were well placed for such activities, such as the caretaker of a church hall where the dances were held, whereas other young people would go to dances when they were on holiday at holiday camps. One elegant and graceful young woman entered a disco dancing competition while on holiday and won first prize (she is one of the group of children brought up since birth out of their own homes).

Holidays

At each age more than two-thirds had had a holiday in the last year (see Table 6.10). At 11 years the holiday was always taken with their parents, and this was the case also for the majority of the young people with Down's syndrome at 21 years; 53% of those with at least one parent alive had been on holiday with them. Almost a third had had a holiday with staff of their day centres or residences. One young woman had gone away with a group from her Further Education college, two on holidays organised by MENCAP or Scope (formerly the Spastics Society), and one very able young woman had been to the United States to a meeting of People First, to which she had contributed.

Only two of the 21 year old controls had had holidays with their parents; the great majority who had had a holiday had gone off with their own contemporaries.

Table 6.10. *Holidays, 11 and 21 years, Down's syndrome and controls (percentages)*

	11 years		21 years	
	DS	Control	DS	Control
None	30	19	15	20
With parents	70	81	42	7
Day centre	N.A.	N.A.	7	N.A.
Other organisation	0	0	34	0
Other relatives	0	0	2	3
Peers	0	0	0	70

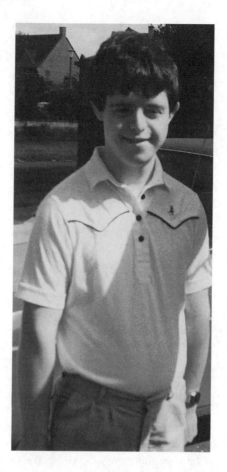

On holiday

Daytime occupation

The day placements attended by the cohort at 11 and 21 years are shown in Table 6.11. At age 11, four-fifths of the children with Down's syndrome (80%) went to schools for children with severe learning disabilities (SLD). One was in the school attached to his long-term residential placement and two attended hospital schools. Two profoundly disabled boys did not go to school at all. Three (7%) high achieving children, a boy and two girls, were at schools for those with mild learning disabilities (MLD); figures in other surveys are 6% (Buckley & Sacks 1987), while 18% (Shepperdson 1984) and about a quarter (Ludlow & Allen 1979) attended either these or normal primary schools. At age 21, almost three-quarters of the young people with Down's syndrome attended either their local day centre or that

Table 6.11. *Daytime occupation, 11 and*
21 years, Down's syndrome
(percentages)

	11 years	21 years
School		
SLD	81	5
MLD	7	0
Residential	7	0
No placement	5	5
Day centre	N.A.	73
FE college	N.A.	12
Farm	N.A.	5
N enjoys it	95	78
Mother's experience		
Easy contact	76	47
Little contact	23	19
Satisfied (at 21)	87	70
Very satisfied (at 21)	66	37

SLD, severe learning disabilities; MLD, mild learning disabilities; FE, further education.

attached to the hospital in which they were living, similar to the 77% and 88% in the Welsh and London studies. In Surrey five young people attended further education colleges; three attended full time, two combined further education with attendance at the day centre. One young woman combined attendance at her centre with a part-time job (hairdressing at an old people's home). Two young men worked on the farm attached to their residential placements. Two young men were still at school and two had no day placement. The circumstances of these last two were very different; one was a very sick young man who stayed at home, almost permanently in bed; the other, who had disliked the day centre he had attended and had been suspended for difficult behaviour, now was the mainstay and support of his mother who had been crippled by a stroke; he ran errands and fetched and carried for her, and on Saturdays worked in his brother's butcher's shop for which he earned £10 (at this time those attending day centres were earning between 50p and £3 per week, often with most of this stopped for meals or snacks). So counting the two in residential placements, the young man working for his brother and the young woman hairdresser, a maximum of four young people with Down's syndrome (10%) were working, all part-time. In contrast, over two-thirds of the non-disabled young people (70%) were in full-time work, one-fifth (20%) were at college or university, two were unemployed and one a housewife.

More than three-quarters enjoyed their day placements (see Table 6.11) though more did so as children than as adults. Only two children were said not to enjoy school; one mother had a rather vague feeling that her (severely disabled) daughter did not enjoy her school and the other, the boy at the school for children with mild learning difficulties, was said to find his school work boring. Most of the adults (78%, compared with 87% in Holmes' study) enjoyed going to their centre (one mother said 'She won't stay home even when she's dying') but one young woman was very unhappy, and in later years flatly refused to attend, and five others went only with reluctance. Getting to their day placements was easy enough for most but nine mothers of the children had problems, all with the special school transport, complaining of the long time the children had to spend on the coach, of unreliability, lateness and long waits – up to an hour twice a day – and of having to go long distances, up to 5 km, to take the children to or collect them from the coach pick-up points. Two mothers, each with two disabled children to take to the pick-up point, had kept their children home, one for three and one for seven months, before it was finally agreed that the transport should come to the children's homes.

> The transport is unreliable and the relief driver comes late – some children can wait an hour. But at least they do now come to the door. We kept [Christine and Tess] home for seven months because the coach wouldn't come here; we had to walk such a long way. We told our MP and he said he could do nothing. I went to the library and looked up the law, and I asked for a home teacher or for transport, so then they agreed that the coach would come to the door.

Two-thirds of the adults (67%) travelled by special transport to the centre, five walked (three of these to the centre in the hospital grounds) and three went by taxi or the family car. Four went by bus or train, three very able young people travelling on their own while one young man was learning to travel independently and was escorted each day on the bus by a 'guide' from his centre. Two families had some problems, one where the coach stop was some way from the family house and the other with the timing of the coach.

> Occasionally the coach is very late and we have to hang about for ages. Then another time a boy had a fit on the coach and they took him straight to the centre so we were left behind.

Over half the children with Down's syndrome (55%) had been in their present school since at least the age of 5 (at which time the 'school' had been a Junior Training Centre, administered by the health authority) and in general there was a good relationship between school and home (see Table 6.11). More than three-quarters of the mothers felt free to contact the school (but less than half the adult centre) at any time, the majority doing so frequently; all but one went to all open days, two-thirds would go at other times as well and a similar proportion would telephone the school if they felt the need. This positive attitude to the schools endured, so that at 21 years only five mothers (15%) said they had been dissatisfied with their child's school and two-thirds said that they had been very satisfied with it. Most, too, were pleased with the placement the young adult attended but fewer, just over a third, were enthusiastic about it. They detailed a wide variety of activities that the young people took part in at the centre – industrial work (12 young people), literacy classes (13), cookery, pottery, sport, hygiene, music, swimming, drama, shopping, horse riding – but four parents commented that the young person had no literacy or educational teaching, three, regretfully, that they did no industrial work.

> She does sport, cooking, washing up, pottery, painting, music. She doesn't do any work. When she was at college they prepared them for going to work. Carla sees what she does now as going back, as if she was back at school.

A few mothers were evidently pleased with the provision for the young person, but many thought more could be done or that the young person was capable of better things.

> He watches videos – mostly war films and *Superman* I think – and does housework and makes coffee and does some reading and writing. He does a bit of industrial work, packing earphones for British Airways. I feel there is something in Roger, he could achieve more in the way of industrial work, fixing things with his fingers. I know it's difficult for them with the cutbacks. He used to go to cafés with them but he hasn't now for months. That's what I hoped they would do for him, train him so that he would be able to do these things independently.

> He does some industrial work and for three years he was in the pottery class. He's definitely gone downhill, he's had no education and no conversation, he hardly speaks when he's there and they can't understand him. I wanted him to have speech therapy but he gets left because he's no trouble. At least now he goes in the education class and he does do some reading and writing and sums.

Friendships

In the account of the children's development until 4 years old (Carr 1975), social contacts for the children – at school, playgroup and at home – were discussed but friendships were not mentioned. By 11 years old, still more by 21, friendships are an important part of any individual's life. We wished

Table 6.12. *Friendships, 11 and 21 years, Down's syndrome and controls (percentages)*

	11 years		21 years	
	DS	Control	DS	Control
Makes friends				
Easily	63	84	61	83
Not very easily	8	16	22	17
With difficulty	29	0	17	0
Has friends				
Disabled	60	16	54	0
Non-disabled	54	100	24	100
None	14	0	22	0
Has a best friend				
Disabled	56	0	37	0
Non-disabled	18	78	2	63
None	26	22	61	37
Has a close friend	N.A.	N.A.	40	73

to know what friendships and social relationships the children and young adults developed, how they felt about them and how the mothers felt about these friendships (see Table 6.12). Nearly two-thirds of both the children and adults with Down's syndrome (like the large majority of the controls) were said to make friends easily. At 21 years this was often a case of the young person being on hail-fellow-well-met terms wherever he went.

> He picks them up; he has a lot of friends round the estate.

> He makes friends with anybody; he gets to know people very well, he'll talk to anybody.

> People I don't know, shop people, will say, 'Hello Andrew'.

These young people were on good terms with all around them, were greeted and recognised, but as one mother said, 'they're acquaintances really, they're friendly, not friends', and there was little indication that the young people had relationships which were close and confiding. Those who had difficulty making friends were equally distributed by sex and covered almost all the ability range apart from those with profound disabilities, for whom the question was not thought appropriate.

Nearly two-thirds of those with Down's syndrome had at least one friend with a disability, many having two or more friends. At age 11, six children with Down's syndrome and at age 21, eight adults had no friend. All at 11 years were very low-functioning children but at 21 the group included two of the most able: one young woman was at this time depressed and withdrawn, and the young man was said to be rather unsociable:

> He's not much of a communicator. Other people greet him, but he doesn't respond. He gets the odd invitation but it's never repeated.

Over half the children, but only a quarter of the adults had a non-disabled friend; most of these were relatives and family friends, but at age 21 one young woman had made friends with people at a church club, one young man with others in his (normal) scout group and another, who lived at home and did not attend a day centre, at the pub he frequented. All but one of the friends of the children with Down's syndrome (compared with only a third of those of the controls) and over half of those of the adults, were from their day placement, school or centre, and it was unusual for them to see each other outside it, although those in hostels would commonly be said to be 'friendly with all his group'. Some mothers commented on the difficulty the young people had in sustaining friendships.

> She talks about four friends that she has at school but they live at such a distance they can never come here.

> She's got lots of friends at the centre but she never sees them outside.

About a quarter of the children in each group were said not to have a best friend, which is similar to the figures given by Newson & Newson (1976) for normal 7 year olds. Most, however, had a best friend, and for the children with Down's syndrome this was most often also a disabled child of the same sex. No fewer than 18% (five boys and two girls, with IQs over the full ability range) were said to have a best friend who was a non-disabled child. The large majority (Down's syndrome 70%; controls 79%) were happy, stable friendships, which had lasted for a year or more.

At age 21, despite their perceived ability to make friends being unchanged, more in each group were now said to have no best friend. In the Down's syndrome group almost two-thirds of the young people had no best friend, and none of these was said to have a close friend. Only one young person with Down's syndrome now had a best friend who was not disabled. Those without a best or close friend included all the six profoundly disabled young people but the remainder had scores at all ability levels, as did those who had friends.

Over two-thirds of the controls visited and were visited by their friends at least once a month but in the case of the Down's syndrome young people, although as already discussed more than three-quarters had friends (see Table 6.12), they saw very little of them at home. Only nine (22%) ever went to see a friend, most being taken to the friend's home by their parents, and only three doing this as much as once a month. Just under one-third were visited by their friends, these being those who themselves visited and some of those with non-disabled friends, but only four were visited as much as once a month. Visits to and from family members were much more frequent but these visits, although seemingly generally enjoyed by the young people, were not necessarily geared to them but were principally family occasions. Lower figures still are seen in the London survey, where none ever visited and only 10% were visited by their friends, although over half visited and were visited by relatives (Holmes 1988).

Teasing and taunting

While friendships are a major positive influence in the lives of most children, teasing and taunting by peers can be a source of acute and long lasting misery. Four of the children with Down's syndrome and nine of the controls were to some extent teased at school. Out of school, however, the figures were reversed; seven children with Down's syndrome (28% of those for whom 'being out of school' was a possibility) and only three of the controls were teased out of school. Asked how their children reacted to teasing, mothers described reactions in the past as well as those to current incidents, so numbers are higher. Around a quarter could cope with the teasing and over a quarter in the Down's syndrome group (but fewer in the controls) were unaffected by it; these were quite able children, their unconcern being by no means likely to be due to unawareness of their situation. The largest number, between a third and half, were upset by teasing and only two in each group reacted aggressively, the children with Down's syndrome concerned being a lively, capable boy and girl who were not generally aggressive.

Asked whether they would try to do anything about the teasing, no control mother said she would attempt any intervention and the same was true of four mothers in the Down's syndrome group.

> He can defend himself now. Once when he was in a paddling pool some children were nasty to him, splashing him. We left him alone. Then he went for them, and it soon stopped.

Seven mothers had intervened in some way; keeping the child in or home from school, speaking to the coach escort or to the school, speaking to the teasing children, or their mothers.

> They get him to do something silly because they think it is funny. I say to them, 'There but for the grace of God go you'. You don't know what to do really. Most of the children around here are not too bad.

> The other kids call out when she is in the garden, 'Look at her, she's mental'. I go round and tell their mothers.

Table 6.13. *Teasing and taunting, age 11, Down's syndrome and controls; age 21, Down's syndrome (percentages)*

| | 11 years | | 21 years |
	DS	Control	DS
Teased, taunted	25	24	56
Teased			
In school	8	24	N.Ap.
Out of school	28	8	N.Ap.
N's reaction			
Unaffected	29	13	22
Copes	21	33	0
Sensitive	36	48	17
Aggressive	14	6	0
Ignores	0	0	17
Not aware of taunting	0	0	44

At 21 years we asked whether those in the Down's syndrome group were ever taunted by outsiders, and if so how the mothers and young people reacted to this (see Table 6.13). Several mothers had not experienced taunting, saying things like 'People are very kind'. Over half, however, had encountered it – staring, sniggering, and remarks – although for two this was now a thing of the past. A third (34%) of the mothers would ignore the taunting or pass it off ('She says, "People are looking at me" and I tell her they are looking at her hair'). Those who responded (66%) were evenly divided between those who would speak to the taunters and those who would shout or glare at them.

Non-responder

When I've taken him on a bus people would say things, not so much about him as about me, things like, 'Why would anyone take someone like that on a bus?' I feel sad, but not resentful.

Responder

You get groups of boys – occasionally girls – who stick their tongues out at her and make remarks. At one time some children from the school up the road would knock on Clare's window and run away, and she wouldn't go into her room for a while. I reported it to the Head and she had the whole school together, and the children did own up. They came round and apologised, and I had them in and gave them a cup of tea and cakes.

Table 6.14. *Awareness of difference, age 21*
Down's syndrome (percentage)

	DS
Aware of self as different	
No	58
Yes	27
Identifies others	15
Reaction to being different	
None known	53
Not bothered	26
Positive	16
Upset	5

Three mothers commented that older people were especially liable to stare, and one that this sort of behaviour could come from an unexpected quarter:

> You get quite a lot from educated people, people we see in museums, who ought to know better.

Almost half the young people were thought not to be aware of the taunting, and only four to be upset by it, the rest either taking it with equanimity or, in two cases, as a joke. In one case this was a highly effective strategy.

> When they laugh at her she laughs with them, and then they get fed up with it and stop.

We asked whether the young people realised that they were in some ways different from other people (see Table 6.14). A fifth of the mothers were not sure, and of the remainder, over half thought they did not realise this. While this group included five of the six profoundly disabled young people, it also included some who were quite able. However, six out of the eight who recognised their difference were amongst the most able young people. One man who did not appear to see himself as disabled nevertheless could see disability in others, e.g., those in wheelchairs, and three young adults identified with other people with Down's syndrome or with other disabilities whom they saw on TV.

> He'll say, 'Oh look, there's someone like me'.

More than half the mothers of the young people thought to be aware of themselves as different had not noticed any reaction to this from them, and a further quarter seemed unconcerned about it. Two able young women took a stronger line, one coming home from her centre with a copy of

Parents' Voice and saying to her mother 'I'm not handicapped!', while the other was even more outspoken:

> She went to a People First conference in the States and she got up on the platform and said 'We can't help it if we're handicapped; we've got our rights'.

Two young people made the most of their status as disabled.

> He knows how to play on it. After dinner he'll sit there and hold his plate out for someone else to take out, or wait for help with his shoes when he can quite well put them on himself.

> She was playing a game with her sister the other night and she wasn't winning and she said to Eve, 'Don't you realise I'm handicapped?'

One young man, however, recognised his disability with distress.

> He knows he's disabled because of his clothes. He can't buy anything and just put it on; they all have to be altered for him. And because he's not doing what we're doing – when he left [Further Education college] he realised that *he* wasn't going to London every day, or having a job.

Sex education and interest

At 21 years we asked the mothers in the Down's syndrome group about the young people's knowledge of sex and interest in the opposite sex. Two-thirds (68%) of the mothers did not know of any sex education the young person might have had; this group of mothers included all those of the profoundly handicapped young people but also many of the most able, and was evenly divided by sex, so the young women had not been made a particular focus in this respect. Nearly a quarter (22%) of the young people had had some sex education at school: two at their day centres (both of them young men living in hostels), and only two, both of them young women, at home. The latter seems especially surprising as sexual matters are of great concern to parents (and were in this group) and it might have been expected that they would make particular efforts to ensure that their sons or daughters were as well informed about sex as was possible. It may be that the mothers felt at a loss as to how they should tackle this subject, a delicate one at the best of times, when they could not be sure how much of their explanation the young person would understand (and parents in Buckley & Sacks' (1987) study preferred sex education to be given at school). Eleven young people (27%), five men and six women, were said to know about contraception; only ten of the young people were said definitely to know that a baby could result from sexual intercourse. None of the young women was on the contraceptive pill or any other form of

Table 6.15. *Sex interests, age 21, Down's syndrome and controls (percentages)*

	DS	Control
Boy- or girl-friend		
Never had one	46	0
Has one	39	71
Had one formerly	15	29
Any serious relationship		
Never	73	7
Yes	27	93
Wants to marry		
Yes	37	48
No	39	52
Too handicapped to express this	24	0
Would like a baby		
Yes	20	46
No	56	54
Too handicapped to express this	24	0

contraception, although one very disabled young woman had been sterilised – her mother had been for some time on the verge of panic about her daughter's sexual safety despite the fact that, with her level of disability, she was always closely supervised. So far there had been only one or two actual incidents to concern this group of parents. One young woman had been taken to a house by two young men she had met in a pub; she left the house the next morning and went to the police station, but, although thoroughly alarmed by the episode, she appeared not to have been molested. Another young woman had engaged in some 'fairly heavy snogging with a lad at her centre who was brighter than her. There's no doubt he used her, but we knew him and she was quite all right. The people at the centre said they'd keep an eye on her but we feel she's entitled to some sexual experience'.

Nearly half the Down's syndrome young people (but none of the controls) had never had a boy- or girl-friend (see Table 6.15); nine of these were very disabled young people of whom it was later said that they were not able to express themselves sufficiently to be able to say, for example, whether they would want to marry or have a child. Twelve young men and ten young women had, or had had, a relationship, all these being with other disabled people, mainly those attending their day centres. Nearly three-quarters of these relationships, compared with only 7% of those of the controls, were said not to have been serious. Over one-third of the young people with Down's syndrome said they wanted to marry and one-fifth that they wanted to have children. This compares with nearly half of the controls in each case (two were engaged and two already married), but, when account is taken of the quarter of the Down's syndrome group who were not able to express themselves one way or the other, the proportions wanting to marry and to have children in the Down's syndrome and control groups are not dissimilar. Indeed, 11 of the Down's syndrome young people, six men and five women, had or had had relationships that were recognised as serious. One young man had become engaged to a young woman and his mother regarded this situation with equanimity.

> Patrick met Sue at the Gateway Club and they have known each other for two years. They have the wedding all fixed up; he has worked out who will give Sue away and who will be his best man – Paul's his best friend but, as Patrick says, he couldn't make a speech, while John would make a splendid speech. So he has decided that Paul could be an usher and John could be the best man. He has bought her a ring – they have exchanged rings. He is devoted to her. Sue's mother was appalled at first but she has come round to thinking it might not be a bad idea. At present we think it would be best if she could go to his hostel and then see how things went from there. He had a long telephone conversation with her the other night and when he came off the telephone he said 'When we are married I will sleep with Sue but I don't want any babies, they cry all night, but Sue says she wants babies.'

In another case the boyfriend was keen to marry the young woman and had spoken to her father on the subject. In six other cases, however, these relationships, although acknowledged to be serious, were discouraged both by parents and staff at the day centres. For one young woman,

> She knows you have to get married to have a baby. It's *the* problem at the moment.

Longitudinal aspects

Health

Figure 6.1 shows that more than two-thirds of those with Down's syndrome were thought at all three ages to have good health (nearly a third of these were rated as very strong). One was consistently rated as delicate. In the controls only two were thought delicate at age 11: both were in normal health at 21, while two others, both women, were now said to be delicate.

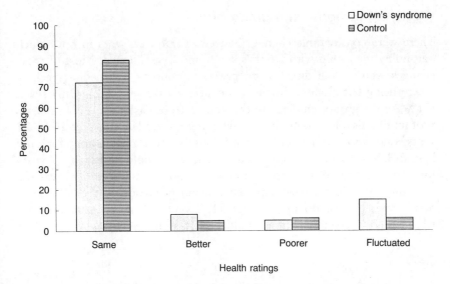

Figure 6.1. Changes in mother's rating of child's health at 4, 11 and 21 years, Down's syndrome and controls. 'Better' indicates steady improvement from age 4 to 21; 'poorer', steady deterioration.

The health of three, two men and one woman, in the Down's syndrome group, and of one in the control group improved over the years, and in two in each group it deteriorated (both in the Down's syndrome group were men and in the controls women). The health of five in the Down's syndrome group and two controls fluctuated, all but one of those with Down's syndrome being thought delicate only at 11 years and the fifth normally healthy only at that time. There was, therefore, little difference between the two groups in consistency of health ratings.

In the Down's syndrome group hospital admissions, having had a serious illness at 11 years, and social class were not related to these findings, but sex was, with women being the more favourably rated: 17 (89%) of the women and ten (45%) of the men were rated throughout as normally healthy (significant at P <0.01). There were three deaths, all of girls, between 4 and 21; one was rated at 4 years as delicate and the two who died at 14 were similarly rated at 11 years. However, if they had survived and been rated as delicate at 21 years the difference between the sexes would still have been significant at P <0.05. It may be, however, that the better health of the women as a group is in part attributable to the loss, through death, of the more ailing females, while men with equally severe ill health live on.

Staying at home and going out

There were considerable changes between 11 and 21 years in how much autonomy the group with Down's syndrome were allowed. Most of these changes were in the direction of greater autonomy for them, especially where being left alone at home was concerned (see Fig. 6.2). Only seven (21%) of the group remained in the same category as at age 11, five being profoundly disabled young people who were never left either at 11 or 21 years, one who was left only for a minute or two and another for only half an hour at each age. One young man, who could be left at 11 years for a minute or two, was now seriously ill and was never left; he was the only one for whom a lower standard of independence on the 'staying at home' measure was obtained at age 21. Twenty-seven (77% of those for whom there was information) could be left alone longer at age 21 than

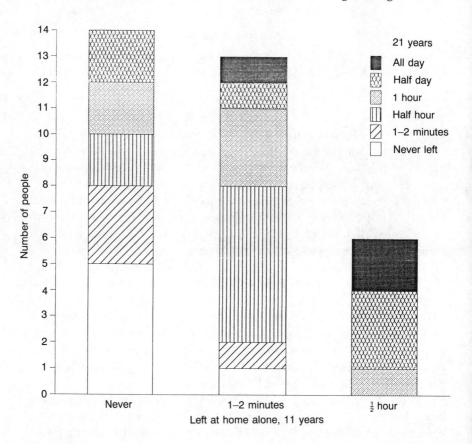

Figure 6.2. Changes in being left at home alone, age 11 and 21, Down's syndrome.

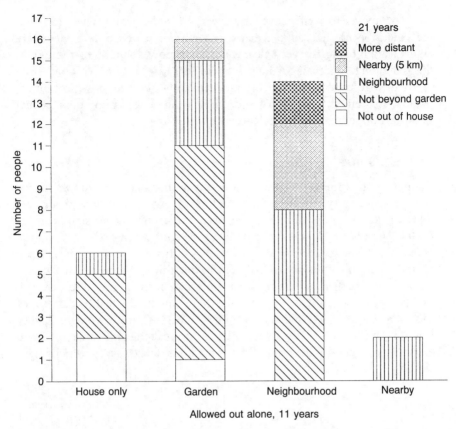

Figure 6.3. Changes in going out alone, age 11 and 21, Down's syndrome.

they were at 11, including four who at 11 could not be left alone at all or only for a couple of minutes, who now could stay on their own for half a day or more.

So, with only a few exceptions, parents felt increasingly able to trust their young people with Down's syndrome in the house alone. The situation is somewhat different when we consider changes in the young person's ability to go out on his or her own (see Fig. 6.3). Just under half (46%) had more freedom at age 21 than they had had at 11, this group comprising mainly quite able young people who, having had some freedom at 11 in their garden and immediate locality, could now go further afield. Two-fifths (41%) of the young people, however, were in the same category as at 11, two-thirds of these (28% of the whole group) being forbidden to venture beyond the garden at either age. While this group included some of the most profoundly disabled young people almost a half (seven) had ability levels of above, to well above, the average for the group. Five (13%) of the young people had slipped back in the amount of freedom they were allowed, one being the very sick young man now confined to the house, the remaining four being young women who as 11 year olds had been allowed to go round their locality independently but were now prohibited, mainly, it seemed, because of the parents' anxieties about their sexual safety, from going outside the garden on their own.

Friendships

Ratings by the mother or carer of how easily they made friends were consistent across the years in just over half the Down's syndrome group and 80% of controls, the difference between the groups being significant at $P < 0.01$ (see Fig. 6.4). Of those rated consistently all but two (6%) in the Down's syndrome group and one in the controls were rated as making friends easily on both occasions. Nearly one-third of those with Down's syndrome were seen as making friends more easily as adults, and one-fifth as having greater difficulty; the former were equally divided by sex but of those having greater difficulty six out of the seven were women. Ability levels did not distinguish between the two groups – mean IQs were 43 and 42.6, respectively – and neither did moving house since age 11, which might

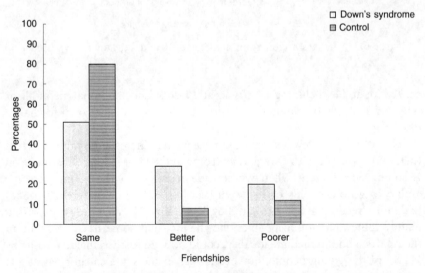

Figure 6.4. Changes in ability to make friends age 21 compared with age 11, Down's syndrome and controls.

have had a disruptive effect; this had occurred for 40% and 42% of the two groups, respectively.

The ease with which an 11 year old with Down's syndrome was able to make friends was not a good predictor of his or her likelihood of having a close or best friend at age 21; 43% of those said at 11 to make friends easily had a best friend at 21, compared with 50% of those who at 11 had difficulty in making friends. Nor was friendliness at age 11 related to having a boy- or girl-friend at age 21: 57% of those who made friends easily and 60% of those who had had difficulty at 11 were said at 21 years to have a boy- or girl-friend. No effect of sex, nor of ability level could be seen in either case.

Discussion

Between the two groups of children and young people, those with Down's syndrome and the controls, many differences were of course found, but there were many areas of life where differences were not as striking as had been expected. The Down's syndrome group were not more often ill than were the controls, although, as Turner *et al.* (1990) also show, illnesses tended to be more serious, especially in the profoundly disabled group. A small number suffered from multiple health problems and very poor health; nevertheless, compared with the controls they did not as a group make excessive demands on family or hospital doctors. Most of those with Down's syndrome, like the controls, maintained good health over time, and in both groups poor health as a child did not necessarily presage poor health in adulthood. However, in the Down's syndrome group significantly more of the women had consistent good health. Since the inception of the study in 1963, eight out of the nine deaths that have occurred have been of females; while it has not been possible to demonstrate that those who died were of significantly lower mental abilities (Carr 1988a), it may be that they were the more vulnerable physically, while men who may have been similarly frail continued to survive. For whatever reason, it does seem that those women who do not succumb may enjoy quite robust health.

Visual, hearing and weight problems, as assessed by their families, were more frequent in the Down's syndrome group as has been found in other studies. Visual problems are found in about half (Buckley & Sacks 1987) to two-thirds (Turner *et al.* 1990; Shepperdson 1992) of study populations, the latter figure being similar to that in the present study. Similar again is the finding that fewer are identified with hearing problems, rates given ranging from 8% to 26% (Buckley & Sacks 1987, Turner *et al.* 1990;

Myers & Pueschel 1991; Shepperdson 1992). However, this low rate may be due to failure to recognise problems that exist (Cunningham & McArthur 1981). A higher figure of 48% has been found in people over the age of 50 (Hewitt *et al.* 1985). The findings of the present study support those of others in showing that more people with Down's syndrome are overweight than are non-disabled people, and that this is more pronounced in females, and tends to increase with age (Buckley & Sacks 1987; Bell & Bhate 1992). This is a probable health hazard for people with Down's syndrome who, like many of those without disabilities, find dieting hard and exercise less attractive as they grow older, and many will need help if they are to counter excessive weight gain. (A simple booklet on healthy eating and exercise, written especially for people with Down's syndrome, is now available (Sawtell 1993).)

If differences in health were less marked than expected, much greater differences were seen between the two groups when independence, range of occupation and friendships were considered. Almost a third of the adults with Down's syndrome could not be left in the house alone for any length of time and over half could not go beyond the garden on their own. At a time when to most young adults freedom and independence are the basis of their lives, the large majority of these young people were confined and supervised in a way that most non-disabled young people do not experience beyond their earliest school days. Quite a sharp distinction is seen between the supervision needed in and out of the home – nearly twice as many parents were happy to leave the young person alone within the home for an hour or more, compared with those who were prepared to allow him or her beyond the confines of the garden and into the streets. As they grew older and more capable the young people were increasingly trusted to be safe within the home, but far less confidence was shown in their ability to cope on their own outside. Despite some parents' fears about a young person's vulnerability to callers, when they were inside the house, perhaps with the door locked and provided the young person could be relied on where cookers, gas fires, stairs and so on were concerned, they were thought to be reasonably safe. Beyond the four walls of the house, or the garden fence, many hazards lay. Danger from traffic loomed large amongst these hazards; when freedom at age 21 was related to the mothers' ratings of the children's traffic sense at age 11, 50% of those who at 21 went far afield, but only 17% of those not allowed out beyond the garden, had been thought to be well aware of traffic hazards at 11. Other possible hazards were the difficulty of finding the way in unfamiliar surroundings, of coping with getting on and off buses and trains, and of being aware of time in order to start the homeward journey early enough; but probably the most important factor, apart from traffic, was the mother's worries about the young person's encounters with other people, from those who at one end of the scale might be no more than rude or unfriendly to those who could pose a more serious threat, with the possibility that the young person might be misled or taken advantage of. These were particularly cogent worries for the mothers of the young women (and may have been at least partly responsible for the four who were more restricted at age 21 than at age 11) but were present too for the parents of the young men. Parents of non-disabled youngsters are fearful of the same dangers, but they have more confidence in the youngsters' ability to look after themselves; in any case they know that these young people will not tolerate restrictions placed upon them. Parents of the disabled young people not only felt a heightened degree of anxiety for the young people's safety, but were also in practical terms more able to impose restrictions. And so restrictions were imposed: the majority of these 21 year olds were accompanied and escorted wherever they went.

Almost all the 11 years olds in both groups went to school, and, although the schools were different in kind, both groups could be seen as engaged in age-appropriate activities. By 21 years a small number in each group were similar in that they attended further education, but for the majority, two-thirds or more in each case, their paths had diverged; the non-disabled young people were in paid employment, the Down's syndrome young people attended their local day centres. Only one, a young woman, was in paid employment (Putnam *et al.* (1988) also found only one out of 30 adults to be in competitive employment), though several more seemed to have the potential for it. With such a wide range of ability in the young people, there was a wide range of activities the parents would have preferred to see them engaged in in their day centres, from more literacy work and daily living skills to straightforward industrial work. Many parents, while appreciating the difficulties the day centres' staff worked under and the value of what was offered, nevertheless felt that there was more their young people could do, achieve and learn if the opportunities allowed.

Leisure activities and interests were fewer and more circumscribed in the Down's syndrome than in the control group, as has been found also in other studies. Putnam *et al.* (1988) note a preponderance of 'passive and non-community-based activities' which they see as similar to the findings for other groups of people with learning disabilities. In the present study, active participation, for example in sport, was no different from that of the controls but community-based leisure pursuits were much more infrequent. Putnam *et al.* (1988) detail a variety of steps already taken in some parts of the United States to increase community integration: for example, integrated recreational clubs, perhaps similar to the PHAB (Physically Handicapped and Able Bodied) clubs in this country, 'pairing' of disabled and non-disabled adults for community leisure activities, etc. However, none of the young people with Down's syndrome in the present study was involved in any such scheme, nor was any mentioned by either Holmes (1988) or Shepperdson (1992). The United Kingdom may lag behind the United States in this respect.

Another major area of difference between the two groups was that of friendships. For non-disabled teenagers and young adults peer relationships become increasingly important but for the young people with Down's syndrome it was a different story. Most had friends, but for many the friendships did not take a central place in their lives; this continued to be occupied by their families and close relations. The difference could be seen most clearly where relationships with a member of the opposite sex were concerned. Nearly half the young people with Down's syndrome were said never to have had such a relationship, and only a quarter, compared with virtually all the controls, to have had a serious relationship. Such relationships were seen by mothers of the controls as inevitable and, furthermore, as almost entirely the young person's own business; they may have worried about these relationships, and might, as an extreme measure, offer counsel but it would have been almost unthinkable that they should interfere with their son's or daughter's love affairs. By contrast, the parents of the Down's syndrome young people monitored and regulated any friendships that seemed likely to go beyond the casual level, the liberal few giving permission for these to continue, the majority actively discouraging them. While this attitude may seem interfering and paternalistic, there was little to suggest that either parents or staff were thoughtlessly domineering. To them the young people lacked the ability to make even the fallible judgements to be expected of any young person; they saw them as vulnerable, and saw it as their job to protect the young people from the most disastrous consequences of any such misjudgements. While in some cases this may have been over cautious, it would be a brave one amongst us who would say they were entirely wrong.

SEVEN

Effect on the families

Families are not static but constantly evolve as the members of it alter. Starting as a couple, most will then experience a profound change in the structure of their lives with the birth of their first baby; further changes take place with the arrival of other children, and with their development from babyhood to childhood to adolescence, each new stage necessitating shifts in the roles, responsibilities and concerns of each family member and, pre-eminently, in those of the parents. These stages are followed by those in which the 'children' become adults and move away from the family home, perhaps to start families of their own. The parents are left to some extent bereft, but they also have the chance, perhaps for the first time in 20 years or so, of consulting their own wishes and following their own preferred pursuits, rather than these being as a rule subordinated to those of the family. All these stages have their advantages and drawbacks – the child who grows beyond the stage of needing to be fed and dressed and bathed now wants a bicycle, worse still wants to ride it on the roads, with all the gut-wrenching anxiety that this entails – but they are seen as the normal progression, observed in and discussed with other families all around. When a child has a disability this normal 'life-cycle' (Farber 1959) is interrupted; the stages are not reached at the usual times, some may never be reached at all. In this part of the study we tried to discover what the effect of these anomalies in the life-pattern had on the families: in particular we wanted to know whether the families were damaged by them, and if so, to what extent.

Learning of the disability

The first impact of the child on the family occurs when they learn of his or her condition. Many studies have been made of how parents were told that their baby was disabled (e.g. Tizard & Grad 1961; Pueschel & Murphy 1976; Murdoch 1983). All the studies are retrospective, some quite briefly (Carr 1970), some asking for the recall of events of 20 years ago or so. These latter studies have always had a question mark over them regarding the validity of the data obtained, and whether the events recalled

119

may have been distorted over time (Ludlow 1980). The present study, in which the mothers were asked at the outset how they had been told of the baby's condition, offered an opportunity to look at these questions. At the time of this first interview, 80% of the babies were aged 6 months or less, three-fifths being no more than 2 months old and no baby being over 2 years. Ten questions were asked: about who had broken the news and to whom (mother, father, or both), the baby's age at the time, whether the news had come as a shock, whether the mother had suspected something was wrong, would rather have been told sooner, or later, whether she wanted a second opinion and if so whether she got it, and whether anything could have been done to make the telling easier. At 21 years the interview was repeated; identical questions were asked, the answers being recorded verbatim in each case. Twenty-nine mothers who had been interviewed on the first occasion were available at 21 years.

The most striking finding was the high degree of similarity between the two records. Across the 10 questions 82% of the replies were essentially similar (albeit with perhaps different wording). The most consistent replies (over 85% in each case) were to questions on who broke the news, who was told, whether the news was a shock, whether they would rather have been told later (all but three on the first and all on the second occasion said they would not), and whether they had asked for and got a second opinion. The least consistent replies (59%) were on the question about whether anything could have been done to make the telling easier, though with no clear trend in the direction of the changes.

It has been suggested that 'memories of the mode of telling may be coloured by feelings which have accumulated through the years' (Ludlow 1980), and it might have been expected that changes in the mothers' recall of the events of 20 years ago would be in the direction of greater bitterness and resentment. This expectation was not borne out. Generally speaking the trend, in the rather small number of discordant responses that there were, was in the other direction. Fewer mothers recalled feeling shocked, or that they would have wished to have been told at a different time or would have liked a second opinion; more recalled that they had recognised the baby's condition for themselves and more that both parents had been present when they were told about it.

Effect on brothers and sisters

Amongst all the distresses parents feel when they are told that their baby has Down's syndrome, one of the most often expressed concerns the possible effect on their other children. While they mourn the loss of the normal

Table 7.1. *Quarrels between sibs, 11 and 21 years, Down's syndrome and controls (percentages)*

	DS (n = 16)		Controls (n = 28)	
	11 years	21 years	11 years	21 years
None	37	81	18	47
Some	44	19	54	21
Many	19	0	28	32

See Table 2.1 for definitions.

Table 7.2. *Index child jealous of sib, 11 and 21 years, Down's syndrome and controls (percentages)*

	DS (n = 17)		Controls (n = 28)	
	11 years	21 years	11 years	21 years
No	94	100	71	82
Fairly	6	0	18	4
Very	0	0	11	14

baby they had expected and face with apprehension the future for the one they have, they are also beset by fears that his or her presence in the family may have an adverse effect on, and may even ruin, the lives of the other children. So it has been a major interest of the present inquiry to try to discover at each stage what has been the impact of the child with Down's syndrome on his or her sibs. We asked about how the sibs got on together, about jealousy, behaviour and health; what the mothers saw as the overall effect of the child with Down's syndrome; and about the future.

Relationships are difficult to predict in families but it was perhaps to be expected, because of the widening gap in interests and abilities of the children with Down's syndrome and their sibs, that personality clashes would be found less frequently between them than in the control families, and this is seen from the data in Table 7.1. At each age, more than a quarter of the children in the control families quarrelled frequently, compared with less than a fifth in the Down's syndrome families at age 11 and none at age 21. It should be noted that, in Tables 7.1, 7.2 and 7.3, those Down's syndrome families in which all the sibs were 7 or more years older (i.e., were aged 18 or more at the 11 year phase) have been excluded, so these findings do not simply reflect a difference in the age gaps in the two groups.

Table 7.3. *Sib jealous of index child, 11 and 21 years, Down's syndrome and controls (percentages)*

	DS (n = 18)		Controls (n = 28)	
	11 years	21 years	11 years	21 years
No	67	100	64	82
Fairly	33	0	18	0
Very	0	0	18	18

It seems that, especially as they grew older, the occasion for quarrelling was less likely to arise where one sib had Down's syndrome.

Similarly, there was less jealousy between those with Down's syndrome and their sibs than in the case of the controls (see Tables 7.2 and 7.3). At 4 years old nearly half (48%) of the sibs of those with Down's syndrome were said to be to some extent jealous of the Down's syndrome child. At 11 years this was true of only a third, and of none at 21. No sib of those with Down's syndrome was said to be very jealous, compared with 18% at each age in the controls. The age of the sib had minimal effects but these such as they were, were in opposite directions in the two groups: 50% (3/6) of younger sibs and 22% (4/18) of older sibs in the Down's syndrome group were rated as jealous, while the reverse obtained in the controls, with 14% of younger and 32% of older sibs said to be jealous. In neither case, however, does the difference approach significance. Where sibs were jealous, the ability of the children with Down's syndrome covered almost the whole IQ range, with only one in the severely and none in the profoundly disabled group, so it did not appear that sibs were more likely to be jealous if the child was more disabled (and therefore perhaps taking up more of the mother's time). The jealous sibs were, however, all (100%) close in age, ± two years, to the child with Down's syndrome, and while this was true also in nine families where the sibs were not jealous, these constituted only half (50%) of this group. So although jealousy was relatively rare in this cohort, it seemed more likely to occur where the sibs were nearer in age to the child with Down's syndrome.

The picture is then of quite harmonious relationships between the young people with Down's syndrome and their sibs, and indeed 90% of the mothers felt that at 21 years they got on well together. Byrne *et al.* (1988) have similar reports, from 72% of mothers of children with Down's syndrome and, two years later from 83%. These support the trend in the present study for amicable relationships between most sibs which get better over time. In the Surrey controls, only 44% were said to have amicable

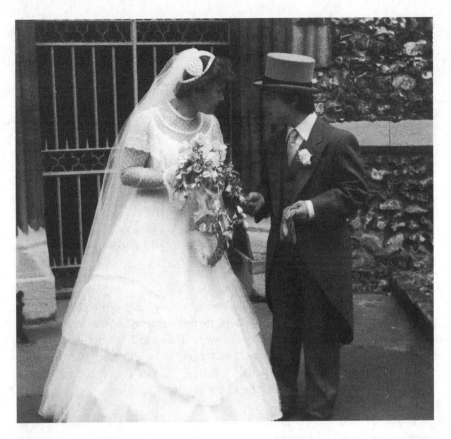

An usher at his sister's wedding

relationships with their sibs, and in over a quarter there were marked problems between them; this difference too, between families with and without disabled children, has been remarked on elsewhere (Byrne *et al.* 1988).

At 4, 11 and 21 years the families were asked about any worries they might have concerning the health and behaviour of their other children, and their replies are summarised in Table 7.4. At 4, over two-thirds of the sibs in each group were seen as easy children who gave no real trouble, and at 11 years this was true for between about half and two-thirds, apart from the controls at 11 when under one-third were rated as problem-free. At 4 and 11 years the higher proportion of problems in the controls was thought perhaps to have been due to the higher proportion of young sibs in these families: at 11 years there were almost twice as many children aged 12 and under in the controls compared with the Down's syndrome group, and more control mothers were concerned about the other children's health

Table 7.4. *Sibs' problems, 4, 11 and 21 years, Down's syndrome and controls (percentages)*

	n	None	Behaviour	Health
4 years				
DS	28	86	14	N.A.
Controls	34	69	31	N.A.
11 years				
DS	23	61	22	26
Controls	36	28	45	49
21 years				
DS	27	52	22	33
Controls	29	62	10	28

Total percentage in some cases exceed 100 as some had problems of both health and behaviour.

(Down's syndrome 33%; controls 61%, difference not quite significant at $P < 0.05$). It may be that the mothers of the controls, without a disabled child to be the focus of their worries, were more ready to notice problems in their other children. By age 21, however, these children had matured and four particularly problematical control families could not be traced, which may also partly explain the lower levels of problems in the controls at this time.

At age 11, for the 18 Down's syndrome and 25 control families with other school-age children, the Rutter A and B scales (Rutter *et al.* 1970) were completed by the mothers and teachers. On the A (parents') scale no sib of a Down's syndrome child scored above the cut-off point but three (9%) sibs of controls did; on the B (teachers') scale four (21%) of the sibs of the Down's syndrome children scored above the cut-off point as did six (18%) of those of controls. There was, therefore, little indication of any greater degree of disturbance in the sibs of the children with Down's syndrome than in those of the controls.

The mothers in the Down's syndrome group were asked at 11 and 21 years, how they thought the other children had been affected by their disabled sib (see Table 7.5). At each age about one-third thought the other children had benefited, and just under half that they had both suffered and benefited, while at age 11, but not at 21, a small number of mothers (four) thought the other children had only suffered from having a brother or sister with Down's syndrome. The difficulties described related mainly to the time the mother had had to spend with the Down's syndrome child, leaving her less, and perhaps insufficient, time for the other children, while three

Table 7.5. *Effect of Down's syndrome child on sibs – mothers' ratings (percentages)*

	11 years (n = 23)	21 years (n = 20)
None	9	20
Caused difficulties	17	0
Brought benefits	30	35
Both	44	45

mothers spoke of teasing, or 'remarks', that the sibs had been subjected to at school. Several mothers, however, remarked spontaneously on their surprise that their other children did not seem embarrassed by the person with Down's syndrome, and that their other children's friends had come freely to the house and had accepted and interacted with him or her.

The following are a selection of the comments made by the mothers, first by those who thought their children had suffered from having the child with Down's syndrome in the family, followed by the comments of those who thought they had benefited.

(Do you think they have suffered?)

11 years

Susan says people stare at us. Neither she nor her brother will take him out on their own; they don't want him.

His younger brother has had to grow up very quickly and become the big brother; he hasn't had enough time spent on him. His sister has been lonelier; if he'd been normal he would have been company for her. As it is she has been virtually an only child.

21 years

They must have done. It must have made a difference, she took up all my time.

He didn't bring his friends home for her [his non-disabled sister] to meet.

At school boys said to Mark, 'You've got a silly sister' and he had a fight over it. It upset him but he put a stop to it. I've never had anything like that myself, people are very good to her.

The benefits the other children were thought to have gained were mainly in compassion, tolerance, and feeling for all people with disabilities, while two mothers felt that through the presence of the person with Down's syndrome family ties had been strengthened and the family kept together.

(Have they benefited in any way?)

11 years

Having her has made the others realise how lucky they are. It's really made no difference to their lives.

They have more awareness of other people's problems and more readiness to accept other disabled people. It's been a broadening experience for them.

21 years

We all have, it's enhanced all our lives; we've gained in understanding and sympathy for other people.

Tom was terribly upset at first; he wanted a sister, but he idolises her now. When he was at home he used to bring in all his friends, and his girl-friends; they were all terrific.

At 21 years we asked about the amount of contact the sibs had with their brother or sister with Down's syndrome and how much they were expected to have in the future. In two-thirds of the families (68%) at least some sibs had a great deal of contact (in nine out of the 19 families there were still sibs living at home), while in 11% they had none (in one family the young woman with Down's syndrome lived away from home and in the other two the adult sibs had moved away). Looking ahead, two-thirds of those who currently saw much of their brother or sister with Down's syndrome, and all of those who saw them little or not at all, were expected to keep in touch with them in the future. Similarly, one-third in each group (30% and 33% respectively) were thought likely to take their disabled sib into their homes when the parents were no longer able to look after them (one young man was already living with his sister and her young family after the deaths of both their parents). So the amount of contact that the person with Down's syndrome had at the time with his or her sibs bore little relationship to expectations about the amount of contact in the future.

There was, however, a strong relationship between social class and whether or not the mother expected that someone else, sibs or other relatives, would take the young person into their home, with a much higher proportion of working class mothers expecting this to happen: 75% of middle class and 25% of working class mothers did not expect anyone to do this (significant at P <0.01).

We asked whether the sibs were worried about their own chances of having a child with Down's syndrome, and whether they had made inquiries, or intended to, about the risks. Sixteen (59%) of the 27 concerned were said not to be worried and in a further six families (22%) the matter had not been discussed. In only four families (15%) were the sibs sufficiently concerned that they had either requested, or intended to request, antenatal diagnosis. In one further case the young woman's sister, although worried, had made no inquiries before the births of either of her two (normal) children.

Effect on the mothers

Mothers' health

At 4, 11 and 21 years, the mothers were asked to rate their own health. The results are summarised in Table 7.6. Between half and two-thirds of the mothers in each group said their health was good, with the proportions falling somewhat at 21 years. Slightly fewer mothers in the Down's syndrome than in the control group reported good health, and rather more that they were depressed, the latter difference being significant at age 11 but not at age 4 or 21. Twelve mothers in the Down's syndrome and 13 in the control group (at 21 years) had had a spell in hospital in the previous ten years, and eight and 11, respectively, had visited the doctor in the previous four weeks. Eleven mothers in each group had had what was judged to have been a serious illness: in the Down's syndrome group one mother had multiple sclerosis, two had had strokes, one had had two heart attacks, three had had major operations (e.g. gall bladder); in the controls, one mother had myasthenia gravis, one cancer, one had had an unwanted pregnancy and had given

Table 7.6. *Mothers' ratings of their own health, Down's syndrome and controls, 4, 11 and 21 years (percentages)*

	n	Good	Depressed	Run down
4 years				
DS	38	58	50	10
Controls	41	63	41	15
11 years				
DS	35	67	39**	35
Controls	37	72	6	22
21 years				
DS	30	50	23	17
Controls	30	59	10	21

See Table 3.4 for significance levels.

Table 7.7. *Means and ranges of Malaise Scale scores, and percent scoring 6+, of mothers of Down's syndrome and controls, at 11 and 21 years*

	DS				Controls			
	n	Mean	Range	Score 6+ (%)	*n*	Mean	Range	Score 6+ (%)
11 years	35	3.5*	0–7	29	37	2.3	0–7	16
21 years	30	4.2*	0–16	23	29	2.6	0–6	10

See Table 3.4 for significance levels.

up the baby for adoption, four had had hysterectomies. Seven mothers in each group had more minor complaints such as asthma, infections and blood pressure problems.

Mothers' ratings of their own health were not related to age, nor whether they were working, nor to IQ, cooperativeness or level of self-help skills of the young person with Down's syndrome at 21 years. However, in the Down's syndrome group middle class mothers reported better health than did those in the working class group (significant at *P* <0.05) and this was significant also for the two groups of mothers combined.

At 11 and 21 years each mother completed the Malaise Inventory (Rutter *et al.* 1970). Mean scores, ranges and the proportions scoring six or more, for both groups, are shown in Table 7.7. Mothers in the Down's syndrome group had higher mean Malaise scores than the controls at both ages, and more had scores of six or more (usually accepted as being outside the normal range – M. Rutter, personal communication), although this latter difference is not significant. As is often found, scores were higher for working class than for middle class mothers, and this was significant at each age for the Down's syndrome group (see Table 7.8) and for the two groups combined (also significant at *P* <0.05).

Since the Malaise Scale has been said, following careful evaluation, 'to provide an appropriate description of stress' (Bradshaw 1982) the findings on this population were examined in relation to a number of other factors which could be related to stress (age of mother, health, occupational status etc.), and to a number of factors connected with the person with Down's syndrome (IQ, academic and self-help skills, personality, independence, etc.). In the Down's syndrome group Malaise scores were higher at both ages for mothers saying they felt depressed, as was also the case for the controls at age 21; whereas only in the control group were scores higher at age 21 for those saying they felt rundown, and at both ages for those saying they felt both rundown and depressed (see Table 7.9). In the Down's

Table 7.8. *Means and ranges of Malaise Scale scores by social class, of mothers of Down's syndrome and controls, at 11 and 21 years*

	DS			Controls		
	n	Mean	Range	*n*	Mean	Range
11 years						
NM	16	2.6	0–7	18	2.1	0–7
M	17	4.4*	0–7	19	2.4	0–7
21 years						
NM	16	2.9	0–10	15	2.4	0–6
M	14	5.8*	1–16	14	3.0	0–6

See Table 3.4 for significance level of NM versus M.

Table 7.9. *Malaise Scale scores related to mothers' health and children's independence, Down's syndrome*

	DS		Controls	
	11 years	21 years	11 years	21 years
Mother				
(a) Depressed	4.85**	6.86*	n.s.	4.67*
(b) Not depressed	2.67	3.43	n.s.	2.39
(c) Rundown	n.s.	n.s.	n.s.	4.17*
(d) Not rundown	n.s.	n.s.	n.s.	2.22
(e) Depressed and rundown	n.s.	n.s.	3.89*	4.12**
(f) Neither	n.s.	n.s.	1.79	2.05
Child	21 years			
(g) Can go out alone	1.73			
(h) Not beyond garden	5.68**			
Good reading skills	$r = -0.61$**			

See Table 3.4 for significance levels: (a) compared, with (b), (c) with (d), (e) with (f), and (g) with (h).

syndrome group, Malaise scores were not related to the mother's general health rating, her age, whether she was working, whether she felt the Down's syndrome person had affected her ability to work, or whether she was lonely. Turning to factors concerned with the person with Down's syndrome, at neither age was the Malaise score related to IQ, personality, manageability, or to any level of behaviour, sleep or health problem, or to whether he or she lived at home or elsewhere. At age 21, however, Malaise scores were higher for those mothers whose young people were more dependent, in that they were not able to go beyond the garden alone, while lower Malaise scores (and better reports of the mothers' health) were associated with better reading skills and, to a lesser extent, with a better vocabulary (see Chapter 3). The association between Malaise scores and reading skills was particularly strong for the middle class group ($r = -0.75^{**}$), while, although tending in the same direction, it was not significant for the working class group ($r = -0.43$).

In summary, in the Down's syndrome group Malaise scores were higher for working class mothers, for those saying they felt depressed, and for those whose offspring could not go outside the garden gate alone and had poor reading skills. No other factors, either in relation to the mothers themselves, or to the abilities or personal qualities of their Down's syndrome offspring, have been identified.

Loneliness

Mothers of children with disabilities are sometimes seen as socially isolated and lonely (Lonsdale 1978). In the present study, mothers were asked whether they thought that having their child with Down's syndrome had made them lonely. At 4 and 21 years one-fifth (21% and 20%, respectively) and at 11 years, 28%, replied that it had. These replies were not consistent across the ages, only two mothers answering affirmatively at all three ages and five at two out of the three ages. (Only two mothers answering affirmatively were lost to the study, both at 21 years.) Two mothers who had said they had been made lonely no longer did so after the child had gone into long-term care, and another who had done so at 4 and 11 years said at 21 that her husband's retirement had improved the situation for her. For those saying they were lonely, mean scores on the Malaise Inventory were higher, being 4.7 at 11 years and 6.2 at 21 years, compared with 3.0 and 3.7, respectively, for the non-lonely group, but, with large standard deviations and only 10 or fewer in the 'lonely' group, the differences do not approach significance. A similar position is seen in relation to the support that the mothers said they had had from friends and neighbours, and from their own families (Table 7.10).

While there is little difference in the level of family support reported (apart from at 4 years), mothers who said they were lonely felt, at each age, that they had had less support from friends, but again small numbers preclude significance. At each age the majority of mothers, about three-quarters, disagreed with the suggestion that the child might have made them lonely, some of them strenuously. Many said that the child him/herself was good company, many that in fact they had made more friends through the child.

Table 7.10. *Loneliness, and support from friends and family, Down's syndrome (percentages)*

	Lonely			Not lonely		
		Much support from:			Much support from:	
	n	Friends	Family	*n*	Friends	Family
4 years	8	12	0	30	40	23
11 years	10	0	20	27	26	22
21 years	6	17	50	24	54	50

4 years

He's brought me a tremendous number of friends; he picks up people.

11 years

I've made more friends, I go to meetings, and sales, and to the school, and we talk over problems and that's helpful.

21 years

She makes me an awful lot of friends. There are terrific compensations.

Some mothers, however, did feel lonely, as exemplified by the following quotation from a mother at 11 years.

You are definitely isolated, particularly round here; people keep themselves to themselves. You're not so conscious of it when they're tiny and in prams but it's harder now, especially when they're discussing their children, you're a conversation stopper. You're even isolated from the other mothers of handicapped children because they are so scattered.

Working mothers

Increasingly over the last few decades mothers have expected to continue working while they bring up their families, or to return to work once their children are old enough. Combining work and a family involves a good deal of often complicated arrangements and adjustments, and it seemed likely that this would be still further affected where the child was disabled. (see Table 7.11). At each age fewer mothers in the Down's syndrome group were working, the difference being significant at $P < 0.05$ at 21 years. A number of mothers in each group at 21 years old had taken retirement because of either age or ill-health; if these are discounted the proportions still working in the two groups are much closer (Down's syndrome 58%;

Table 7.11. *Mothers working, 11 and 21 years, Down's syndrome and controls (percentages)*

	DS		Controls	
	n	%	n	%
4 years	38	34	41	41
11 years	38	55	37	68
21 years	30	37	28	64*

See Table 3.4 for significance levels.

controls 69%). Most mothers in both groups worked part-time: the numbers working full time in the Down's syndrome group when the child was 4, 11 and 21 years old were – one, two and one, and in the controls – two, four and five. However, eight out of the 11 mothers in the Down's syndrome group (at age 21) who were working felt that their ability to work had been affected by the young person with Down's syndrome. This was almost always because of the restriction on the hours they were able to put in, which were governed by the hours of the day centre the young person attended; while in some cases this also restricted the kind of job the mother was able to take. Seven more mothers had given up work because of the needs of the young person, so that, in all, the ability to work was, or had been, adversely affected in half the mothers in the Down's syndrome group. In contrast, only three mothers (14%) said their husbands' work had been affected, while all of the eight fathers seen at the interviews said that it had not been so.

Effect on the marriage

When the young people were 21, each mother was asked to rate her own marriage on a scale from 1 ('very good') to 5 ('poor'); and those with a Down's syndrome child were asked what had been the effect of the baby's birth on the marriage (see Table 7.12). Almost half the mothers in each group rated their marriages as 'very good'. A sizeable proportion (27%) of the mothers in the Down's syndrome were widows, and it was thought possible that they might, looking back, have taken a more positive view of their marriages than would women who were still living with their husbands. A separate analysis of the responses of the widows, however, showed that they too rated the marriage as very good in half the cases, so the original finding is not biassed by the replies of this particular group.

Table 7.12. *Quality of marriage, and effect of child with Down's syndrome age 21 (percentages)*

	DS	Control
Quality of marriage	(*n* = 27)	(*n* = 26)
Good	48	54
Mostly good	48	35
Average	4	11
Effect of child at birth	(*n* = 29)	N.A.
None	48	
Good	14	
Bad	28	
Bad at first, then good	10	
Divorced (omitting Catholics)	(*n* = 34)	(*n* = 32)
	9	19

Nearly half felt that the arrival of the baby with Down's syndrome had not affected the marriage, but over a quarter felt that it had. Five mothers, including two who later had become divorced, felt that their husbands did not give them the sympathy and support they needed at this time; three that the baby had effectively put a stop to their sex lives because of anxieties about possible future pregnancies and about contraceptive methods.

> It didn't make any difference to our feeling for each other but it finished our sex life. I went to the Family Planning Association but I was very scared of conceiving and eventually it affected my husband.

One mother was jealous of the attention her husband gave the baby, but four said that the baby had brought the couple closer together.

> At first it made things very difficult, we couldn't work out which of us had failed. As he [the Down's syndrome child] got older, after he was about 4, or 5, it drew us together.

Three marriages in the Down's syndrome group (7%) had ended in divorce, as had six in the controls. In the Down's syndrome group there were 11 Catholic families, in whom divorce would have been very unlikely. If these families are discounted, the divorce rate for the remaining 34 families is 9%, just under half that for the controls. In the Down's syndrome group marital status was known, either currently or at least until the child died, for all the families apart from one who emigrated when the child was 3 years old. However, nine control families, who had been intact when they were last seen, could not be contacted at later ages and their circumstances are not known. If all these families, only one of which was Catholic, had remained intact (and some at least had shown signs of marital discord before contact with them was lost) and if they were included to make the total number for the controls up to 37, the proportion divorced would be 15%. Thus, even when the best possible state for the controls is assumed, their divorce rate would still be somewhat higher than that for the Down's syndrome group.

Social life for the mothers

Going out

At all ages (15 months, 4, 11 and 21 years) the mothers were asked how much they were able to go out, with their babies or children, or on their own, or with their husbands or other escort. These ratings were combined, taking the most favourable rating at each age (i.e. that in which the mother said she went out most often) to provide an overall score. The proportions going out rarely or never, sometimes or often at each age are shown in Table 7.13. (Regrettably, at 11 these questions were omitted for the control mothers.) For each age for which there are data, mothers in the Down's syndrome group were going out less often than were the controls, and this difference is significant at 15 months and 4 years. At 21 years, ten mothers in the Down's syndrome and 20 in the control group (33% and 69%, respectively) went out very often, once a week or more, and this difference too is significant at P <0.01 (and in the Down's syndrome group could not be explained by either age or social class[†]). Nevertheless, nearly two-thirds at 11 years and over three-quarters at 21 went out often (once a month) or very often. As was found at 4, two-thirds of the mothers in each group felt they went out as much as they wanted to, or that they could go out more if they chose to.

> We could easily go out more. I suppose we've got out of the way of it; when we do go out we sometimes wish we hadn't.

Of those saying at 21 years that they would like to go out more, all in the Down's syndrome group (and 7/10 in the controls) were going out once a month or more, and were evenly divided between older and younger mothers (over or under 57 years). Asked what prevented them from going out as much as they would like, a wide variety of reasons was put forward – constraints of a job, housework, illness, or 'inertia'. Financial problems

[†] Mean age of the mothers in the Down's syndrome group who went out very often, often, or seldom or never were 57.4, 58.1 and 57.1, respectively: the proportion of middle class mothers who did so were 31%, 50% and 19%, respectively, and of working class mothers, 36%, 36% and 28%, respectively.

Table 7.13. *Mother going out, 15 months, and 4, 11 and 21 years,*
Down's syndrome and controls (percentages)

	n	Rarely/never	Sometimes	Often
		Mother went out		
Down's syndrome				
15 months	35	43**	23	34
4 years	36	36*	22	42
11 years	34	15	23	62
21 years	30	3	20	77
Controls				
15 months	32	3	28	69**
4 years	32	9	28	63
21 years	29	10	7	83

See Table 3.4 for significance levels.

were cited by nearly a third (29%) and problems to do with the person
with Down's syndrome by just over a fifth (21%).

So, compared with the controls, going out was more restricted for the
mothers in the Down's syndrome group when the children were young, the
gap between them narrowing as the children grew older. Factors which
might have been expected to contribute to this, such as the presence of the
person with Down's syndrome in the home, or the age of the mother, did
not seem to have had a major influence, while those who wanted to go out
more were those who already went out a good deal. It seems that out-of-
home activities, and the wish for them, may be governed more by personal
than by situational factors. In order to explore this, the relationship
between wanting to go out more and Malaise scale scores, and feeling
depressed and rundown, were examined. Mothers in both groups who
wished to go out more had slightly higher mean Malaise scores (4.4, compared with 3.9 for those not wishing to go out more), and were slightly
more likely to report themselves as depressed and/or rundown (43%, compared with 26% of those not depressed/rundown). However, the differences are small and, even for the combined groups, not significant. The
paradox remains in which some who are often engaged in out-of-home
activities would have liked more than they had, and some who seemed
relatively restricted were content with their lot.

Holidays

Over two-thirds of the mothers had had a holiday in the previous year (at
age 4, within the previous four years) with barely any differences between

Table 7.14. *Holidays, 4, 11 and 21 years, Down's syndrome and controls (percentages)*

			Yes	
	n	None	With N	Without N
Down's syndrome				
4 years	39	8	92	N.A.
11 years	36	28	72	N.A.
21 years	30	23	57***	20
Controls				
4 years	40	5	95	N.A.
11 years	37	19	81	N.A.
21 years	29	21	10	69

See Table 3.4 for significance levels.

the two groups (see Table 7.14). By 21 years, over half the mothers had been on a holiday without the young person. However, at 21 years, 17 mothers in the Down's syndrome group, but only three in the controls, had had a holiday with their son or daughter, either in addition to or instead of a holiday on their own; this difference being significant at P <0.001. Families with a disabled young adult still seemed to feel responsible for taking him or her away on holiday, while this was very much a rarity in the non-disabled group.

Support from friends and relatives

We asked the mothers about their friendships, and about how much they saw of friends and family; and at 11 and 21 years, how much help those in the Down's syndrome group had had from them (see Table 7.15). Forty

Table 7.15. *Help from friends and family, 11 and 21 years, Down's syndrome (percentages)*

	Friends		Family	
	11 years ($n = 37$)	21 years ($n = 29$)	11 years ($n = 36$)	21 years ($n = 29$)
None	24	17	22	17
Some	27	14	31	14
Much	22	42	22	55
No help but supportive	27	24	22	14
No help needed	0	3	3	0

per cent in each group said they had few friends (one mother in each saying she had none); the remainder saying they had many or very many friends. Around four-fifths saw their own grown-up children at least once a month (Down's syndrome 79%; controls 86%) with about half seeing them weekly. Fewer saw their other relations (the parents' brothers and sisters, etc.,) as often as this, with half seeing them only occasionally (Down's syndrome 37%; controls 41%) or never (Down's syndrome 21%; controls 7%), and less than a quarter seeing them weekly (Down's syndrome 21%; controls 14%).

About half the mothers at 11 years, but less than a third at 21, said they had had little help from their families, and the same was true of their friends. About a quarter said they did not feel they needed help, but most added that their family or friends were supportive, accepting and taking an interest in the child and being friendly or talking to him or her.

11 years

They've offered to pick her up off the coach in the evening but I haven't availed myself of it.

He's always welcome in their homes.

21 years

My sister will always have Annie to stay, although there's no need now. She would rather have Annie; she's so much easier than the other two [non-disabled children].

They're still our friends; they haven't deserted us.

One mother spoke of a less friendly neighbour.

She kept on about how she was worried that the value of her property might go down.

A composite score was derived from the 21 year ratings of the help mothers had had from family, friends and neighbours, and this was related to scores on the Malaise scale. There was no evidence that low levels of support were related to high Malaise scores (indicating greater stress); on the contrary, the relation between high support and high Malaise scores just failed to reach significance at $P < 0.05$.

Longitudinal aspects

Because of small numbers, made even smaller in this part of the study by losses from death not only of the individuals with Down's syndrome but also of their parents, it was advised that no longitudinal statistical analysis was possible. Consequently only simple comparisons across ages have been carried out.

Effect on the sibs

For those in both groups who were seen at all three ages (4, 11 and 21) the proportions of the sibs who were causing anxiety because of their health, behaviour or both (only behaviour was asked about at 4) are shown in Table 7.16. At 4 years, only three mothers in the Down's syndrome and five in the control group said they were having trouble with the child's sib(s). In the Down's syndrome group, all three were still in the same position at 11 years and two out of the three at 21; in the controls, four at 11 and two at 21 were still causing concern. From 11 to 21, for those families represented at both ages, changes for better or worse (i.e. from some to no trouble reported, or vice versa), together with figures for those in which there was no change, are shown in Table 7.17. In three (14%) in the Down's syndrome and four (14%) of the control families problems of health had been exchanged for those of behaviour, or vice versa, thus taking the percentages to 100 in each case.

Table 7.16. *Sibs' health and behaviour problems, 4, 11 and 21 years, Down's syndrome and controls (percentages)*

	DS (n = 22)			Controls (n = 28)		
	4 years	11 years	21 years	4 years	11 years	21 years
None	86	73	46	82	29	64
Health	N.A.	18	27	N.A.	29	29
Behaviour	14	9	18	18	21	7
Both	N.A.	0	9	N.A.	21	0

Table 7.17. *Consistency and change in sibs' problems, age 11 to 21, Down's syndrome and controls (percentages)*

	DS	Controls
n	22	28
No change	54	22
Better	0	50
Worse	32	14
Problem exchanged	14	14

Table 7.18. *Consistency and change in sibs' relationships, age 11 to 21,*
Down's syndrome and controls (percentages)

	No change	Better	Worse
Relationships			
Down's syndrome (*n* = 16)	50	44	6
Controls (*n* = 21)	21	58	21
Jealousy: N of sib			
Down's syndrome (*n* = 17)	94	6	0
Controls (*n* = 28)	64	25	11
Jealousy: sib of N			
Down's syndrome (*n* = 18)	67	28	5
Controls (*n* = 28)	61	25	14

In 12 families in the Down's syndrome group no change was reported,
10 reported no problem at any age, and two mothers spoke of continuing
problems of health or behaviour. Fewer control families showed this consistency but over half, compared with none in the Down's syndrome group,
reported improvement at 21 years. Fewer control families found things
becoming more difficult at 21, but the difference, represented by seven families in the Down's syndrome group and four in the controls, is not significant. Where there were more problems, most were due to the emergence
of health problems (Down's syndrome, 5/7; controls, 3/4). There was then
no significant difference between the groups in the persistence of health
problems in the sibs.

At age 11, three sibs of controls had scored above the cut-off point on
the Rutter A (parent) scale, and six sibs of controls and four of the Down's
syndrome children, on the B (teacher) scale. At 21, three of these control
families were no longer in the study, and the parents of one Down's syndrome man were dead, so there was no information on his sibs. Of the
remaining four families of controls and three of Down's syndrome young
people, none now expressed concern about the behaviour of their offspring;
one control and all three families in the Down's syndrome group said they
had no worries about the sibs. Numbers here are very small, but, such as
they are, they do not suggest that disturbance is more long-lasting in the
sibs of those with Down's syndrome than in the sibs of non-disabled
children.

Relationships between sibs tended to improve as they went from childhood to adulthood, especially in the controls (see Table 7.18). Jealousy of
a sib was expressed by only one child with Down's syndrome at age 11
and this had resolved by 21; however one-third of the non-disabled sibs

Table 7.19. *Consistency and change in mothers' views of the effect of the child with Down's syndrome on the sibs, age 11 to 21 (percentages)*

	11 years	21 years
None	11	22
Caused difficulties	11	0
Brought benefits	39	28
Both	39	50

were jealous of the Down's syndrome children at 11 but by 21 this, too, was mostly a thing of the past. In the controls, jealousy was more equally expressed between the index child and his or her sibs, and some lingered on into adulthood. Thus, although the presence of a disabled child in the family might be expected to occasion greater jealousy on the part of the other children, (and many mothers felt they had spent overmuch time with the child with Down's syndrome, which might have been expected to lead to resentment on the part of the other children) in this sample there was little difference from that found in families without a disabled member, at least as perceived by the mothers; what there was tended similarly to diminish over the years.

Changes in the views of the mothers as to the effect the child with Down's syndrome had had on the other sibs were examined in relation to the 18 who were seen at both 11 and 21 years, shown in Table 7.19. Half of the mothers seen on both occasions did not change their views; most (4/9) saying that there had been both difficulties and benefits. Just over a quarter (28%) had become more positive, moving towards seeing either benefits or no effect where previously they had seen problems, while just under a quarter (22%) had moved in the opposite direction. Overall, then, time had not produced a major shift either way in the mothers' views on this topic.

Effect on the mothers

Mothers' health

Of the 29 mothers in the Down's syndrome, and 28 in the control group, who were seen on every occasion at 4, 11 and 21 years, one-third (34%) in the Down's syndrome group, and just over a half (54%) in the controls, rated their health similarly each time. Most of these (Down's syndrome 70%; controls 73%) reported good health on each occasion, these constituting 24% and 39% of their respective groups as a whole. Seven (24%)

mothers in the Down's syndrome group and three (11%) in the controls gave reports of their health improving over the years, and seven and four, respectively, reported worsening health, while for the remaining five and six mothers the reports fluctuated. Two of those in the Down's syndrome group whose health was better by 21 years were mothers of profoundly/ severely disabled young men now living away from home, although that had also been the case at 11, when both had rated their health as poor. Three more mothers reported better health at 21 despite having been widowed since the previous occasion. Three of those reporting worse health had experienced serious illnesses, one a severe stroke, one arthritis and a third multiple sclerosis, while another had had a series of operations. Those in the Down's syndrome group who reported worsening health were on average nine years *younger* (age 51) than were those reporting better health (age 60), so the older age of the mothers in the Down's syndrome group is unlikely to have been a determining factor in their experience of worsening health.

No characteristic of their Down's syndrome offspring could be found which was associated with the mothers' poorer health: the son of one was profoundly disabled, another a difficult young man, and another was in long-term care, but the remainder were easy, pleasant young people. Furthermore worsening health was not clearly related to the mothers' feeling run-down or depressed: five mothers said they were neither, one (whose son was in long-term care) felt she was both, and one (who had had a stroke) that she was depressed.

Overall, therefore, about three-fifths of the mothers in each group (Down's syndrome 59%; controls 64%) reported health that was either unchanged or improved over time, while less than a quarter (Down's syndrome 24%; controls 14%) found their health deteriorating. Once again, the findings are more adverse for the Down's syndrome group, but the differences are small and non-significant and there is little to suggest that deterioration in the mothers' health could be ascribed to factors connected with the child with Down's syndrome.

In the Down's syndrome group, better health in the mother when the children were 4 years was associated with their being able to work by the time their offspring reached 11: 62% of those mothers in good health, compared with 42% of those with poor health at 4 years were working at 11 years (significant at $P < 0.005$). At 11 years, mother's health was not associated with working by 21 years (possibly because, of those still in the study at 21 years, eight were over the age of retirement). Neither association was significant in the case of the controls.

Correlations between the Malaise scale scores at 11 and 21 were significant for both groups (Down's syndrome: $r = 0.51**$; controls: $r = 0.72***$),

Table 7.20. *Mean Malaise scores, and number of scores of 6+, for mothers lonely at 11 or 21 years, or both, by social class*

	NM			M		
	n	Mean score	Number scoring 6+	*n*	Mean score	Number scoring 6+
11 years	7	3.1	1	7	6.9	6**
21 years	8	2.9	0	5	9.2	4**

See Table 3.4 for significance level of NM versus M.

showing greater stability in the controls. The scores of six mothers in the Down's syndrome group increased by three or more points (two by three, one by four, and one each by six, eight and nine points), while four had decreases in this range (two of three, and one each of four and seven points). In the controls, there were only two changes of this magnitude, being decreases of, in one case, three and in the other, four points.

Looking at Malaise scores in relation to loneliness over time, of the 17 mothers who at any time, at the 11 or 21 year stage or both, said they had felt that the child had made them lonely, mean Malaise scores were 5.3 at 11 and 4.9 at 21, somewhat above the general means of 3.5 and 4.2, respectively. More striking are the differences in the figures when these are broken by down by social class (see Table 7.20). (Two mothers in the (M) working class group were lost after 11, and one (NM) middle class mother who had not completed the Malaise Scale at 11 did so at 21). The figures in the table are in accord with those in both this and other studies, showing that mothers in working class groups were at greater risk of stress; in this population this has now been shown to be clearly associated with loneliness.

Going out

In the Down's syndrome group, there was a steady increase in the number of mothers going out often (see Table 7.13), so that the significant difference between the Down's syndrome and control groups at 15 months, in those who went out once a month or more, was not evident at 4 years, although there was still a preponderance of mothers in the Down's syndrome group who seldom went out. By 21 this too had disappeared, the only difference now remaining being the higher proportion of the controls who went out once a week or more. The same progression over the years, from few to more outings, was not seen in the control group, two-thirds of whom already at the 15 month stage were going out to an extent not exceeded by the mothers in the Down's syndrome group until after 11. Among individuals, 16 mothers in the Down's syndrome, but only five in the control group, went out more over the years; four and 14, respectively, remained the same (all but one in the Down's syndrome group going out often at each stage), three and two, respectively went out less, and the remainder fluctuated.

These figures show, firstly, that the mothers of babies with Down's syndrome were more tied than were those in the control group, despite many (over two-fifths, Carr 1975, p. 85) having ready-made baby sitters in their other, older children; and, secondly, that as the children with Down's syndrome grew older the mothers became more able to go out, although it might have been expected that it would be more difficult to get sitters for these larger children, especially if the older sibs were no longer available. It should be noted that the increased freedom of the mothers in the Down's syndrome group is not attributable to the number whose offspring had moved away from home: only one of these featured at 11 (his mother is one of those who rarely went out at this time) and even if the six at age 21, five of whose mothers went out often, are discounted, the proportion going out often is almost unchanged at 75%.

Holidays

Four mothers in the Down's syndrome group had had no holiday on two occasions; two at 4 and 11 years, and two at 11 and 21. One of the latter was the single mother of a profoundly disabled young man but the other three were mothers of capable, pleasant individuals; all four were from working class families. In the controls, one mother had had no holiday at 4 or at 21.

Help from friends and family

A total of 26 replies (out of a possible 59) were consistent across the two occasions, the largest single category being the seven mothers who said at both ages that they had had much help from their families (see Table 7.21).

Table 7.21. *Consistency in help from family and friends, age 11 to 21 (numbers)*

	Help given			
	None	Some	Much	Not needed but supportive
Friends	3	3	3	3
Family	3	1	7	3

In the remaining ratings, 24 were of more and nine were of less help. The ratings for friends and family were combined, and this composite score was compared at 11 and 21 years to see whether, overall, mothers were reporting more or less help over the years. Leaving aside the five whose ratings did not change, 16 indicated more and five less help over time, the difference being significant at $P < 0.05$ (McNemar's test, $P = 0.047$). Broken down by social class the figures for those reporting more and less help were: NM, more = 7 and less = 5 (n.s.); M, more = 9 and less = 2. So, while there was a general trend towards more help being experienced as time went on, it was particularly pronounced in working class mothers. This was not a case of their catching up over time: the mean composite score for the working class mothers was higher at both 11 and 21 years (NM, 2.7 and 3.2; M, 3.3 and 4.7). Hence, working class mothers reported more support from family and friends and saw this as increasing more over the years.

In summary, findings in respect of the sibs of the two groups changed little over time: those in families with a Down's syndrome child 'grew out of' health and behaviour problems to much the same extent as did those of the controls; jealousy faded away rather more completely for those in the Down's syndrome group. The health of the mothers ran a similar course in the two groups, and where that of the Down's syndrome mothers deteriorated, this could not be ascribed either to their age, to depression, or to characteristics of their Down's syndrome young people; better health, until they reached retirement age, was associated with future employment. Few mothers, at any one age, complained of feeling lonely but overall this affected about half the group, and was associated with stress in mothers in the working class group.

Discussion

Telling the parents

The investigation of the mothers' descriptions of how the news of their babies' condition was broken to them, first very soon after this event and then approximately 20 years later, has shown a very high degree of consistency between the two accounts. Two possible explanations for this consistency have been put forward (Carr 1988a): one, that the strong anxiety that accompanied the telling was responsible for the retention of the memory of it, as has been shown in other studies (Walker 1958); and two, that this retention was due to reiteration, the mothers having recounted or rehearsed the event many times over the years. Whatever the reason, the mothers remembered with considerable accuracy how they were told of their babies' condition, and this conclusion is supported by two other reports. Gath (1985b) followed up 22 mothers of surviving children with Down's syndrome who had been interviewed soon after the birth of their child; they were interviewed again between eight and nine years later when 'the similarity of the accounts is marked'. Cunningham *et al.* (1984) re-interviewed 12 parents, originally seen within three weeks of disclosure, two years later when 90–100% of replies were in agreement with the earlier interviews. The impression that many workers have remarked on, that this event stays vividly in the mothers' minds, seems by and large to be true. Further, there is no evidence overall of resentment building up over time. If a mother expressed resentment 20 years on, it was usually because she had felt it at the time. The more common finding, also reported by Gath (1985b) was that, if anything, resentment dissipated. There seems, then, to be little reason to be concerned that studies of this topic that are carried out long after the event will result in grossly distorted data, or that they will contain an exaggerated loading of negative feeling.

The effect on brothers and sisters

The study of the effect on the sibs suggests that they do not suffer major disadvantages from the presence of the Down's syndrome person in the family. Certainly, some mothers felt that their other children had suffered, but these were balanced by the, somewhat larger, number who thought they had benefited. Quarrels and jealousy were rather less than in other families, and the longitudinal results support the prediction of Byrne *et al.* (1988, p. 40) that relationships would improve over time. Byrne *et al.* (1988), who also identified, in a younger group, better relationships between sibs in families with a child with Down's syndrome than in families of non-disabled children, suggest that this might come about either because children with Down's syndrome are less volatile and thus less likely to be drawn into confrontations, or because the sibs of children with Down's syndrome are encouraged by their parents to be more forbearing with the Down's syndrome child. To these hypotheses may be added the suggestion that, especially as they grow older, areas of interest may become more and more discrete between the disabled and non-disabled siblings, and this too might reduce the likelihood of conflict. That being said, it should be remembered that all the data in the present study, apart from those from the Rutter A and B scales, are derived from the mothers' reports and from how they saw the situation for their other children (and there is evidence of the fallacy of assuming that parents can answer adequately for a child, particularly where experience of stress is concerned – Yamamoto *et al.* 1987).

Nevertheless, the findings are generally in agreement with those of studies of the sibs themselves (Hart & Walters 1979; McConachie & Domb 1983; Boyce *et al.* 1991), which have shown the brothers and sisters to be predominantly positive in their attitudes to their disabled sib and not themselves unduly burdened. Nor, in the present study, were there other signs of distress, such as a higher rate of disturbed behaviour in the sibs; what there was tended to diminish over time in a way that was similar to (but if anything more pronounced than) that seen in the families of the controls.

Despite the weight of the evidence, from this and from other studies, *against* the proposition that children are harmed by having a sib with Down's syndrome, about half the mothers felt that their other children had suffered. Few could point to any hard facts about this, and the views they expressed seemed to derive from an uneasy intuition, exemplified by the comment given by two mothers: 'They *must* have suffered.' That this is true of only a small number, and that most sibs do not suffer undue disadvantage, should be publicised far more widely than has happened until now, in order to ease at least some of the heartache endured by new parents of babies with Down's syndrome. In the words of Abramovitch *et al.* (1987), 'It should be a relief to parents faced with the prospect of bringing a Down's syndrome infant into the family to hear that it is possible for the child to get along with the siblings in a normal fashion.'

Effect on the mother

Where the mothers were concerned the situation was different. There were indeed areas in which the mothers in the Down's syndrome group experienced no more difficulties than did the controls. Few (around a quarter at any one time) felt they had been made lonely by having a disabled child, and they went out increasingly as their children grew older (even if not as much as did the controls). Little difference was seen in the mothers' ratings of their marriages, while the divorce rate was at least no higher in the Down's syndrome than in the control group. Other studies of the effect of a disabled child on the marriage have given conflicting results, some suggesting adverse effects (Friedrich & Friedrich 1981) and others little or no effect (Waisbren 1980). Looking only at those studies concerned with children with Down's syndrome, Byrne *et al.* (1988) rated 28% of the marriages in their sample as good and 7% as poor or very poor; the figure for poor/very poor marriages from a sample of families with non-disabled children was 24% (Richman, Stevenson & Graham 1982). In another longitudinal study of families with a Down's syndrome or a non-disabled child, by 8 years old there had been three divorces in the Down's syndrome and one in the control group, and there were no significant differences in ratings of the quality of marriage (Gath & Gumley 1984). In a later paper (Gath & Gumley 1986b), fewer marriages in the Down's syndrome group were found to have ended in divorce (5%, compared with 16% in families with a child with other forms of learning disability), although there were no significant differences in the quality of marriages where the parents were still together. Higher divorce rates have been quoted for families of older people with Down's syndrome, i.e., 24% (Holmes 1988) and 19% (Shepperdson 1992), but there are no comparative data apart from Holmes' report of 27% divorces in families of people with autism. Differences in methodology and definitions notwithstanding, the conclusions drawn from these studies are similar. Despite the fears that have been expressed about the deleterious effects of a disabled child on marital relationships, there is little evidence that a child with Down's syndrome is more likely than any other to lead to disruption of the family.

Nevertheless, there were areas in which the mothers in the Down's syndrome group were at a disadvantage. They were less able to go out to work than were mothers in the control group, and, while this difference between the groups was small during the childhood years, this changed as they grew older, becoming significant by the time they were adults, as has been found also in other studies (Baldwin 1985). At this time, for most parents, their children have left home or are sufficiently independent not to need a constant parental presence in the home, and, the economic climate permitting, mothers can take up employment and work what hours they choose. Mothers of disabled young people are restricted to working limited hours that have to be rigidly adhered to, and this in turn limits the kind of job they can take and the financial and job satisfaction to be gained from it. Unless day centres can extend their hours, or other facilities can be developed that would cater for people with learning disabilities after the centres close (and realistically there is absolutely no immediate prospect of either coming about), mothers will continue to be disadvantaged in their work opportunities if they continue to look after a person with learning disabilities at home.

The mothers in the Down's syndrome group went out less, especially when the children were very young, but even at 21 years fewer, compared with the controls, were going out once a week or more. Many more had taken their adult child on holiday with them; whether this should be included under the label of disadvantage is open to question but it seems reasonable to suppose that many older parents might prefer, when they were on holiday, not to have to consult the needs and wishes of younger people but to do whatever they themselves felt inclined to do. About a third in the Down's syndrome group, as in the controls, wished they could go out more than they did, and this is consistent with reports from other studies (Buckley & Sacks 1987; Byrne *et al.* 1988). However, only 15% of those interviewed by Byrne *et al.* (1988) attributed their difficulty in going out to the presence of the Down's syndrome child, similar to the 21% in the present study.

Having a disabled child had clear effects on the well-being of the mothers. Their health was somewhat less good, rather more reported being depressed, and they showed more signs of stress in that their scores on the Malaise scale were higher and more had scores of 6+ than were found in the control group. Mothers of disabled children have commonly been found to have higher scores on the Malaise scale (Tew & Laurence 1975; Bradshaw 1980; Carr *et al.* 1983). While this might seem too obvious an outcome to need research attention, it has been less simple to show what are the factors responsible for it. In the present study we searched for factors, both those relating to the mother herself (age, employment, etc.) and those relating to her child with Down's syndrome (IQ, self-help and other skills, behaviour disturbance, etc.), that might be associated with stress. However, the only significant results showed Malaise scores to be higher in mothers who said they felt depressed, and at 21 years, for those whose young people were unable to go out independently and, who had poorer reading skills; the latter especially in middle class mothers. A major finding was the association with social class, working class mothers having higher Malaise scores at both ages, and at the 21 year stage poorer health.

Other studies have also focused on parental (usually maternal) stress and what are the factors associated with it. In general, more stress has been shown by mothers with high neuroticism scores, who lack a car, and whose children have behaviour problems (Turner *et al.* 1991). Holmes (1988) found more stress in mothers who had, and were taking medication for, psychiatric problems, who were worried about their health, depressed or run down, and, in only those mothers whose Down's syndrome adult lived at home, where the adult had behaviour problems. Stress in the form of psychiatric disorder, where the marriage relationship was good, was associated with behaviour problems in the child – the same effect was not seen where the marriage was rated as moderate or poor (Gath & Gumley 1986b). Finally, more stress was reported by mothers in working class groups (Gath & Gumley 1986b) and with lower levels of educational achievement (Byrne *et al.* 1988). Moreover, measures taken earlier of behaviour and health problems in the child, and of social class, were efficient predictors of stress, with those in working class groups, whose children had behaviour and health problems, likely to have higher levels of stress four years later (Turner *et al.* 1990). In families of children with a variety of learning disabilities, social class was more closely related to Malaise scores than was the severity of the child's disability (Ferguson & Watt 1980).

To summarise the findings from the different studies, the most consist-ently found associations with maternal stress are other indicators of neur-oticism, problems of health and behaviour in the child (though neither was seen in the present study) and social class. Studies of physically disabled children and their families have shown stress in the mother to be associated with the mother's *perception* of disadvantage, such as feeling socially restricted or dissatisfied with her housing, rather than to objective measures of these factors, such as numbers of outings or levels of housing provision (Carr *et al.* 1983). A similar process was noted by Holmes (1988) in famil-ies of learning-disabled adults. Bradshaw (1980) having failed to find 'really independent variables' associated with stress scores postulates that stress might be 'determined by internal factors, the physiology and personality of the mother'. Some mothers are probably particularly vulnerable, while others are constitutionally better able to shoulder the burdens placed upon them. It will be important to find ways of identifying those who have the greater needs and to ensure that these are met.

One of the most interesting, and surprising, findings is the paucity of associations between maternal stress and factors connected with the child. Studies that have sought a relationship with disability level, as shown by mental testing, have failed to find it (Holmes 1988; Hanson & Hanline 1990; Turner *et al.* 1991). Hanson & Hanline (1990) found a relationship, in the families of their, very young (all under 5 years), group, between stress and low levels of adaptive behaviour but this was not confirmed in families of adults (Holmes 1988), while only poor independent mobility (and read-ing skills) showed a relationship in the present study. To the lay observer it seems axiomatic that a learning-disabled child, i.e. a child with impaired general intelligence, must by that very fact alone be a source of stress to the parents. The evidence shows otherwise. It is not impaired intelligence as such that is stressful, but some manifestations of it, especially impaired competence and difficult behaviour. Although unexpected, these findings should engender optimism. Efforts to boost intelligence levels have met with equivocal success, but competence can be enhanced and behaviour problems modified. It is to these ends that the interventionists of tomorrow should strive.

Finally, social class has been shown, both in this and other studies, to be a major factor in families' experience of stress. Families in working class groups, who are subjected to poverty, unemployment and deprivation, have been shown repeatedly and powerfully to suffer particularly severely from the presence of a disabled child, for all the love and warmth that they afford him or her. A strong case can be made for extra financial and social support for such families, to enable them to cope as well as possible with their disabled child, and to continue to enjoy their own lives.

EIGHT

Help from services

R esilient and resourceful as the families with a child with Down's syndrome are, they do carry a disabled member and they do have special needs. A variety of services exist in this country, as in most developed countries, to meet these needs, but it is a topic of continuous debate as to how far the needs are met and what else should be done. We asked the mothers about their experiences of a range of medical, educational, financial and social services, which ones they had received and what they had thought of them. Some services, such as those from family doctors and health visitors, had been available from the beginning, while others had become available or appropriate only as the children grew older.

Continuing services

Family doctors

An important potential source of help, on hand since the babies' earliest days, is the family doctor. Later, families would learn about other agencies but at first they naturally turned to their GP. At 4, 11 and 21 years we asked how satisfied they had been with their contacts with him or her (see Table 8.1). When the children were 4 years old more than half the mothers had found their family doctor helpful, in that he or she came to see the child and, in many cases, took a special interest in him or her. At 11 years and again at 21 over 70% were happy with their GP, the large majority of these (80%) saying they were very satisfied.

11 years

He's been marvellous; he willingly filled in the form for the attendance allowance, and for him to go to [a holiday home]. It makes life more bearable.

He's known her since birth, and before – she was to have been born at home. If he meets me out he always asks me how she is.

Table 8.1. *Satisfaction with family doctor, at age 4, 11 and 21 (percentages)*

	4 years (n = 36)	11 years (n = 36)	21 years (n = 30)
Not satisfied	44(43)	25(27)	23
Mother fairly satisfied	22(30)	36(33)	23
Mother very satisfied	34(27)	39(40)	54

Figures in brackets at 4 and 11 years indicate proportions for those still in the study at 21. See Table 2.1 for definition.

21 years

We've had the same GP since she was born. I've only got to ring and he'll come out, even at night.

Where the GP was not seen as helpful this was often apparently because of insensitivity or, perhaps, poor training.

11 years

He tells me not to worry about her; she won't live long; I should love the other children.

He won't visit her, even when she had bronchitis. I ring up and they give a prescription over the phone and won't even look at her.

21 years

He's very good in other ways but he doesn't understand Philip.

Over time there was a shift from about a third of the families at 4 years, to more than half at 21, who found their family doctors helpful, and conversely from about two-fifths at 4 who were dissatisfied with them, to less than a quarter at 21. It is a matter of speculation whether this is due to changes in the families, i.e. whether when their children were small they had greater needs and expectations of their GPs, which were difficult to meet, and that this moderated as the children grew up; or whether doctors are now better trained and more adept in their dealings with families of disabled children. In support of the latter proposition is the finding by Byrne *et al.* (1988) that 48% of families of 2–10 year olds saw their GP as very helpful and only 25% as very unhelpful. These figures, derived from families of children with Down's syndrome whose mean age was 5, and who were born 10–17 years after those in the present study, indicate greater satisfaction and less dissatisfaction than in the Surrey study at either 4 or 11 years old. It does seem, therefore, that GPs may be becoming more adept in their dealings with families of disabled children.

Table 8.2. *Saw hospital doctor, at age 4, 11 and 21 (percentages)*

	4 years (n = 38)	11 years (n = 37)	21 years (n = 33)
Never seen	51	70	41
Seen once a year	16	14	32
Seen twice a year or more	33	16	27

Hospital consultants

When they were babies almost all the children with Down's syndrome (82%) had to attend a hospital for check-ups. By age 4 this had reduced to just under half (49%), two-thirds of whom attended every 3–6 months, the rest annually (see Table 8.2). At 11 only 30% attended hospitals at all, roughly half of these attending six monthly or more, and the rest annually. Seven of the 11 who still attended had cardiac problems (as had 7/30 who were not attending hospitals) and by age 21 two had died. At 21, 59% of the young people were seeing a hospital doctor, about half of these (27% of the whole group) seeing the doctor twice a year or more. The doctors seen represented a variety of specialties – psychiatry, thoracic, cardiac, ENT (ear, nose and throat), and orthopaedic and general surgeons.

When the children were 4, nearly two-thirds (62%) of the mothers found their hospital visits unhelpful, complaining of being given little information or advice, and of long waiting times for brief interviews. At age 21 this position was reversed, with 75% of those attending satisfied or very satisfied with their hospital visits. This may have been because by 21 the visits were for a particular purpose that was relevant to the particular individual, rather than, as at 4, for general check-ups, and the mothers who at the 4 year stage felt the visits were 'just a waste of time' may now have felt that more was being effectively achieved; or, once again, it may have been due to an increase in the expertise of the doctors and in their awareness of the mothers' needs.

Health visitors

Health visitors are an important resource for mothers of young children, and at 4 years old their visits were welcomed by two-thirds of the mothers of the children with Down's syndrome, especially where they could give practical help and advice, e.g. on feeding (see Carr 1975). At 11, two-thirds (64%) had not seen a health visitor since the child had started school, and only a quarter (25%) had seen one within the last six months (see Table

Table 8.3. *Satisfaction with health visitor, at age 4, 11 (percentages)*

	4 years (n = 37)	11 years (n = 28)
Not satisfied	3	21
Mother fairly satisfied	27	21
Mother very satisfied	70	58

8.3). Again the views of those who had seen a health visitor were generally positive or non-committal.

> She was very nice; we got on fine. She started a play group here for the mentally handicapped children under five.

Those who were less enthusiastic said, as they did at 4 years, that the health visitors lacked the specialist knowledge that was needed, which in some cases seemed to make them shy away from the family.

> They were very sweet and worthy, and tried so hard to help but their advice just doesn't apply to you.

> They did pop in all right; they were friendly, but as soon as they see what she is they lose interest.

National Society for Mentally Handicapped Children (MENCAP)

Sixteen mothers (41%) at the 4 year survey were members of the National Society for Mentally Handicapped Children (NSMHC) and another nine said they wanted to join. By 11 years only two had dropped out, while three of those who had said at 4 that they wanted to join had done so (as also did the foster mother of one child). So membership was sustained among those interested early on, but none of the mothers who had been disinclined at the start had joined the Society later. At 4 membership was slanted towards the middle class, 68% of whom belonged to the Society compared with 15% of working class mothers (difference significant at

Table 8.4. *Membership of MENCAP (percentages)*

	4 years (n = 39)	11 years (n = 31)
Member	41	42
Wants to join	23	0
Not a member	36	58

P <0.001), but by 11 the figures were 50% and 35%, respectively, and the difference was no longer significant.

Services at age 21

A range of services were inquired about at 21, some of which had not featured earlier. Mothers were asked which services they had been in contact with and how satisfied they had been with them, on a scale as follows:
1, 'very dissatisfied';
2, 'mostly dissatisfied';
3, 'neutral';
4, 'mostly satisfied';
5, 'very satisfied'.

Table 8.5 shows the numbers who had received each service and how satisfied (ratings 4 and 5), neutral (3) or dissatisfied (1 and 2) the mothers were with it. Three groups of professionals (physiotherapists, behavioural psychologists and community nurses) had hardly impinged on the mothers in this group, having been seen by none, two and three people, respectively, and will not be considered further.

Generally speaking, levels of satisfaction were high, two-thirds or more of the mothers being appreciative of all professionals except two – speech therapists and pre-school assessment workers (I will return to these). More mothers were satisfied with the schools their children had gone to than with the day centres, and this was seen more strikingly where those very satisfied was concerned, being 64% and 37%, respectively. This was despite the fact that this group of children, over half of whom had started 'school' by the time they were 4 years old, had gone first to Junior Training Centres run by the health authorities, which became schools only when

Table 8.5. *Satisfaction with services, at age 21 (percentages)*

	n	Dissatisfied	Neutral	Satisfied
School	33	18	0	82
Day centre	27	22	8	70
GP	33	24	6	70
Hospital doctor	18	11	11	78
Social worker	24	8	13	79
Speech therapist	17	17	24	59
Chiropodist	9	0	0	100
Dentist	30	3	3	94
Optician	25	16	4	80
Pre-school assessor	7	28	28	44

these children were 7 to 8 years old. The parents' memories of the schools, and of the further education colleges that some went on to, were predominantly positive.

It was excellent; they took so much trouble and the children were so happy. I can't say enough for them.

There were, nevertheless, criticisms, consisting of comments about poorly trained teachers, an unchallenging curriculum, of ideological disputes, and of the shortage of male teachers.

I thought the more able pupils should have one to two hours a day of proper school work but the Head said that would disadvantage the less able ones.

The boys weren't catered for; they were all women teachers, and there was nobody to play football with him.

In this last case the situation was resolved when the boy went into long-term care in a large hospital where, perhaps ironically, his mother was better pleased with his education: 'The hospital school is very progressive.' In other cases there were, as may happen in any part of the educational system, clashes of personality, with children miserable under one teacher and blossoming in the care of another.

Many parents were apprehensive about the move from school to day centre, and some were, in the words of one mother, 'relieved and delighted' at how things turned out, and especially appreciative of the personal qualities of the day centre staff. Some, however, saw the centre regimes as limited ('They're left doing Lego a lot of the time') and were disappointed by the fact that there was so little prospect of a normal working life, which at the time, was taken for granted by most young people of that age. One mother was appreciative but prophetic:

They do their best under difficult circumstances; I won't like it in a few years' time, the way the cuts are going.

Medical services were highly valued, and, as with other specialties such as social work, this was partly for the professional expertise and the help that was given, but almost equally important was the relationship, for good or ill, that the doctors made with the mothers.

Les had all this bowel trouble and Dr W. gave him a colostomy. But then his bowels functioned and the colostomy was reversed, but of course Les was scarred. When he had to have his appendix out his tummy was so covered with scars that they didn't know where to cut. They rang Dr W.; he was on holiday but he came back to do it.

We see Dr C., he's very nice and concerned; I feel I can talk to him.

> We saw this psychiatrist, a trendy young man who treated me like just a silly mother. I didn't want to see him again.

Opticians and dentists were also highly valued, in the case of the first perhaps because the work that opticians did was usually successful in correcting visual difficulties, and this resulted in a real benefit to the individual with Down's syndrome. Dentists had been consulted by almost all the young people. People with Down's syndrome have a higher rate of both dental abnormalities and dental disease (Barden 1985), but in the past few dentists had much experience of people with learning disabilities and a visit to the dentist was an occasion for mothers to dread. The very high regard in which the dentists were held in this study is a tribute to not only the technical but also the inter-personal skills that the profession seems to have developed.

Social workers were well-regarded and much liked as a rule ('She phones every month and I know I can always phone her') but their lack of specialised knowledge, the difficulty of getting hold of them, and frequent staff changes made for dissatisfaction.

> She was always so busy and it was hard to get hold of her. I always got an answering machine and then she didn't ring back. It wasn't very helpful.

> They're very pleasant and would come if I needed them, but they didn't have a lot to offer. They do seem to change a lot; if you got the same one twice you were lucky.

The two groups given the smallest vote of confidence in this study were the speech therapists and those responsible for assessing the child before starting school, usually a psychologist or doctor. Where speech therapists were concerned the mothers felt that their children did not get enough input and that what they did get had very little effect. Byrne *et al.* (1988, p. 107) note that where a professional provides an intervention designed to help with the child's development, and the intervention is not effective, parental criticism is likely to focus on this disappointing outcome. In the case of pre-school assessment, only seven mothers remembered this event, so individual dissatisfactions might weight results unduly (but only nine had dealt with chiropodists, who got 100% satisfactory ratings). Criticisms of the assessment occasion stemmed from what the mothers saw as a brief, unsympathetic session with, often, a not very skilful professional and little effort made to allow the child to do him or herself full justice, the assessment leading to what seemed to have been a pre-determined outcome – placement at the Junior Training Centre.

Looking at overall satisfaction, 33% of the mothers were satisfied with all services, lower than the 48% found by Byrne *et al.* (1988). In view of this, the ratings for each mother in the present study were combined, and these combined ratings were examined to see whether a 'grumble factor' could be detected – whether there were mothers who were dissatisfied with all services. However, although, as already stated, a third of the mothers were satisfied with all services, no mother was dissatisfied with all. Satisfaction was somewhat higher in working class than in middle class mothers: eight of the 11 mothers who were satisfied with all services were from working class families, and mean scores on the satisfaction scale were 3.9 for middle class mothers and 4.3 for working class mothers. However, the figures do not reach significance and indicate only a trend. Satisfaction was not related to Malaise scores, whether analysed for the whole group or by social class; the tendency was in the opposite direction from that expected, with higher Malaise scores for those expressing more satisfaction with services, but again the differences are not significant.

Short-term care

At age 4 only two children had spent any time in short-term care (see Table 8.6). Nearly a third (32%) of the mothers had been offered it but almost two-thirds (62%) did not know, at that time, that anything of the sort was available. By 11 over a third and by 21 40% had had some short-term care; by 21, however, four young men, who had previously made use of the facilities, were in residential care, and if they are included the figure at 21 rises to 47%. Only one mother at 11 would have liked to have been offered the facilities, five had refused them, and the remainder were neither offered nor had wanted them. Two mothers had tried a number of homes until they found one they were happy with: one took her daughter out of a home because of misgivings about the fire precautions, and one who had been pleased with the children's home her son went to was dismayed by the adult placement ('The doors were always open and people were in and out all the time; it wasn't safe'). The main reason for accepting care was to give the mother and the family a break, but in one case this misfired:

Table 8.6. *Use of short-term care, age 4, 11 and 21 (percentages)*

	4 years (*n* = 37)	11 years (*n* = 38)	21 years (*n* = 30)
Never used	95	63	60
Once/twice	5	26	17
3–4 times	0	3	3
5–6 times	0	8	3
7+ times	0	0	17

I took it up once because I thought it would be nice for the other children, but they were horrified and missed him dreadfully. We never did it again.

More than half the families had never, over the 21 years, used short-term care facilities, nor had they ever wanted them. As regards the possible explanations for families using or not using the facilities, there was no indication that they were more used where the child was more severely disabled: mean IQ for users was 45.9 and for non-users 47.5 (many of the severely or profoundly disabled were in long-term care and their IQs are not taken into account in these calculations), nor were users markedly more difficult than non-users. Age and social class did not differ significantly between the groups, although mean Malaise scores were slightly higher for users (4.7 compared with 3.7 for non-users). It seems that use of short-term care, for those who did not need long-term care, may have been determined mainly by the social needs of the families and by how acceptable they felt the care offered was for their young person.

More help wanted

At 4 and 11 years the mothers were asked whether they would have liked more visits than they had had and the majority said they would not. Only seven (19%) said at each age that they would have liked more visits, three answering affirmatively on each occasion. Only one middle class mother (at 11), compared with a total of 10 working class mothers, would have liked more visits. Asked whether they would have liked more help, and if so what kind of help, about half at 4 and 11 and over a third at 21 could not think of anything they would have liked (see Table 8.7), and by 21 the greatest need was felt to have been for more help when the child with Down's syndrome was younger. For most, the help wished for was, understandably, for more help for the mothers themselves, but Table 8.8 shows that there was a shift over time towards wanting more help for the person with Down's syndrome.

Table 8.7. *Help wanted, age 4, 11 and 21 (percentages)*

	4 years (*n* = 38)	11 years (*n* = 37)	21 years (*n* = 29)
No	47	49	38
Yes			
Now	0	24	10
Previously	53	16	38
Both	0	11	14

Table 8.8. *What help would have been liked, age 4, 11 and 21*
(percentages)

	4 years	11 years	21 years
None	47	49	38
Help for the mother	31	27	23
Help for the child	22	24	39

The largest single category of help, mentioned by eight mothers at 4 and seven at 11 (but only three at 21) was that of help in looking after the child, 'for a few hours, or an evening, or a whole day', to give the mother a break. This was seen as distinct from the short-term care that was on offer, and pre-supposed standards of care that they had not so far experienced.

11 years

I need a break but I can't let her go into the hostel, not even for a holiday, in case she gets ill. The hole in her heart gets bigger every time she's ill.

21 years

She was always ill and I was always sitting here nursing her. I felt stranded; I thought they could have done a bit more to help me. Now it's really much easier, especially with my husband [now retired] around.

Help with housework and more sympathetic dealings with doctors were each wished for by two mothers at the 4 year stage; while at 11 help with housing and early counselling for themselves would each have been liked by two mothers, and better allowances by three.

After help in looking after the child the next biggest category of help wished for, by five mothers at 4 and six at 11 and 21, was more advice and information on how to bring up the child.

4 years

I wanted more information on how she would develop, practical help, not just people telling you not to worry.

11 years

I would have liked to have known about behaviour modification right at the beginning; the course at [a special unit] was the making of me.

21 years

What I wanted was a psychologist I suppose. He used to throw things, and the health visitor suggested tying things in a soft sock that he could throw. We did that but it wasn't any good because it didn't make a satisfying crash.

Three mothers at 4 years and two at 11 wished that earlier teaching, before school, had been available, two for better play facilities for the children, and one for more suitable clothing for her overweight 11 year old son. At 21 years, the principal categories of help wished for were, in the early days, advice on how to help the child, and currently, advice on adult life, sex and employment.

> Our health visitor was very good when she was little but what we need now is information about sex and about her future.

> We'd love to have someone come to see us and help her get a job.

Allowances at age 21

All the young people living at home, apart from two very capable young women, received the Attendance Allowance; nine got the higher rate (given where the disabled person needed attention at night as well as by day) and 18 the lower rate. Two of those getting the lower rate had had the higher allowance in the past, one until she moved into residential care at the age of 20, the other until she was reassessed at 17 years old and the allowance was down-graded, although she was very similar to others who continued to get the higher rate. Only two families had applied for the Mobility Allowance, one being refused and the other accepted; this latter was a very severely mentally and physically disabled young man, but the other, even more multiply disabled and non-ambulant, did not get the mobility allowance. All of those living at home, except the profoundly disabled young man just mentioned, received one or more allowances in addition to the Attendance Allowance; 17 (61%) got the Non-Contributory Invalidity Payment, eight (28%) the Severe Disablement Allowance, and seven (25%) Supplementary Benefit (percentages add up to more than 100 because three young people were in receipt of more than one allowance).

The total allowance individuals living at home received at this time (1985) varied widely, from £28.50 (for one of the capable young women) to £80 per week (for the severely disabled young man who had succeeded in getting the Mobility Allowance). The average total allowance was just under £50 (£49.94) and two-thirds (68%) received between £40.60 and £55.15. Broadly speaking the more severely disabled were receiving, as is intended, higher allowances than the less severely disabled, but there were anomalies; for example, there were the two young men of whom the more severely disabled was receiving £30 per week less than the other, and of two other, almost identical, young men one was receiving £20 per week more than the other.

From the mothers themselves came a strong sense of the part played by happenstance in the allocation of allowances. Twelve mothers (39%), equally represented in the middle and working class groups, had been given no advice on what they were entitled to, although others had been given information by the child's school (nine mothers), their doctor, social worker or MENCAP (three each) or by social services (two). For 12 mothers this advice was sufficient but for others the information that led to allowances being obtained came from a variety of sources – friends, relatives, articles in magazines, the Citizen's Advice Bureau, and, for almost a quarter (23%) from casual acquaintances such as 'a friend at the riding centre', 'a lady I met at music therapy', 'a woman with a child with spina bifida'.

Some mothers, especially of the more competent children, had been reluctant to apply for allowances ('Jenny's too good; I didn't think I'd get it') or felt they should not have them ('I didn't think I really needed it; I feel a bit guilty about taking it'), but others had had stern battles.

A sister who now has her brother with Down's syndrome living with her and her family commented:

> I applied for the mobility allowance because Brian is frightened of buses, he needs both hands to help him on and off and I can't manage that and the two little ones. And he doesn't like escalators or stairs with no back to them, so I'm very limited where I can go. But I was turned down. I appealed, and we had to go up to [town] and Brian was very distressed and could hardly move when they asked him to walk. But they still turned me down.

Two mothers had applied for the higher rate of the Attendance Allowance.

> I didn't get it at all at first. The doctor had the form and asked the questions and I kept saying 'No, no' to them, and I said, 'But these aren't the right questions', and he said, 'Well this is the form I have to fill in'. So I wrote to them telling them what he was like; that from the time he went to school, about 5 or 6, he had this projectile vomiting at night; he had so much mucus, and I'd come back from a party and find it all over the bed and him and the carpet and the walls. I got it straight away.

> When I first applied, when she was 8, I was turned down. I appealed, and had another visit from another doctor and got the full allowance. Then at 16 she was reassessed – did we go through it! We had a great tussle, and I was given the lower rate. Things were no easier, how could they say anything had altered? I appealed, and got another doctor who slanted the questions in a slightly different way; I got the full rate, and went on getting it until she went away [into residential care].

Discussion

Services for families with a child with a disability are intended to make the parents' difficult task easier and more manageable (though in an ideal world they would ensure that the child could lead a life that was equal to that of his non-disabled contemporaries). Overall, this aim was achieved in most cases for most parents, as has been shown also in other studies. Using the same research approach, similar levels of satisfaction with the services they received were found for most professionals in the study of London mothers (Holmes 1988), though fewer were pleased with their social worker (40%) and chiropodist (69%), and slightly more with the speech therapist (70%). Byrne *et al.* (1988) finds satisfaction levels that are somewhat lower than in the present study (although the research methods and criteria may have been different). The highest levels of satisfaction expressed by the mothers of these younger children (for those professionals under inquiry in both studies) were for the social worker, speech therapist, GP and psychologist. Parents in the Welsh study (Shepperdson 1992) were much less satisfied (47%) with the day centre the young person attended, and clearly standards may vary from one part of the country to another. Despite differing levels of contentment with the day centres, some of the reasons for satisfaction were common to the studies, such as the good atmosphere of the centres, and the fact that many of the young people loved going to them; while dissatisfaction was commonly expressed about the limitations of the programmes followed, and the lack of opportunities for and encouragement of work. Many parents, as Holmes (1988) also finds, regretted the absence of contract work, which, when it was available, gave their young people a feeling of working and of going to work each day as did most of the rest of the population; even the educational programmes running in many centres seemed no substitute for that.

Medical and paramedical services were valued on two main counts: firstly, for what they were able to do for the young person, and for the improvement that they brought about for him or her; and secondly, for the professionals' ability to relate to the young person and to the mother (or other members of the family). Family doctors have a particularly important part to play because they are there, in a position of authority and of perceived wisdom, from the beginning. Even if they are not especially interested in or well-informed about Down's syndrome, they should be able to point the mother in the direction of the information she needs, notably from the parent associations.

Health visitors and social workers were well liked and in some cases became family friends. This was more likely to happen where the family was in contact with the same worker over a considerable period, but this was often impossible because of staff changes. While some departments have well-organised systems of hand-over to new workers, this can falter, or, in a climate of financial stringency and staff reductions, no new worker will be allocated. Lack of expertise, which resulted in mothers feeling they gained very little from well-meaning visits, was a serious problem, one that has been noted elsewhere (Byrne *et al.* 1988; Holmes 1988) and one that needs to be addressed. With all the different varieties of disability, some of which, even with a relatively common condition such as Down's syndrome, any one worker will encounter only rarely, no health visitor or social worker can be expected to be *au fait* with them all. Some degree of specialisation, however, with one member of a department at least aware of where to go for information (in the case of Down's syndrome, to the Down's Syndrome Association), would go a long way towards meeting parents' needs.

Mothers who had difficulty in contacting their social worker would eventually give up trying, when it seemed that the worker supposed that she had no urgent needs, and contact would be lost. In other cases, mothers felt that, because they coped well and did not complain about their situation, workers assumed, without asking them, that they did not need help and left them to get on with it. The most intractable difficulty probably comes about when through financial pressures there are not enough services or service personnel to go round the clients, when workers may indeed be thankful not to seek out needy clients. Holmes (1988, p. 413) notes 'a certain sympathy' for social workers who cannot offer the services they know are needed because they do not exist, but are still in the front line between the families and the authorities responsible for the services. Nevertheless, it is necessary to make it clear where services are inadequate, and to bring this home to those responsible for them.

When mothers were asked whether they wanted more professional visits most said they did not, possibly envisaging further intrusions on their time and little likelihood of benefit for themselves. Many, however, could think of help they would have liked. Few wanted more financial support, but some form of 'baby-sitting', to allow the mother time on her own out of school hours, was much wanted, especially when the children were young. Shepperdson (1992) remarks that in her survey parents seldom wanted anything new, rather more or improved versions of what was already available; a baby-sitting service has, however, rarely been provided. Where it has been, as part of services geared specifically to parents' needs (Brimblecombe 1979; Bose 1991) parents have been warmly appreciative of the provision and have given clear evidence of the benefits they derived from it.

The short-term or respite care services were intended to have the same effect, that of giving relief to families, but were not seen in the same way by the mothers, who were adamantly refusing short-term care when the child was 4 years old, the time when they were wishing for some 'baby-sitting'. Byrne *et al.* (1988) found only 14% of families of 2–10 year olds using short-term care facilities, although these included foster families. In Wales use of short-term care increased from 14% of families of 9 year olds to 37% for those in their mid-twenties (Shepperdson 1992), similar to the figure given by Holmes (1988). In the present study, the trends are very similar, with minimal use when the children were small and increasing use over time. It may be that as they get older the young people are seen as less vulnerable than they were as children, and as better able to cope with being away from home, and much may depend on the quality of the service offered, and how confident in it the mothers are. As already mentioned, some individual schemes, where provision is closely tailored to individual needs, have been well received by the families (Burden 1980; Bose 1991).

The other category of help most wished for was advice on how to handle and bring up the child. Again it seems that such advice was not readily available, that where it was the mothers did not know about it, and that service providers were not aware that this was what the mothers wanted. Where such help has been available there is evidence, albeit anecdotal, that parents welcomed this (Cunningham 1987). As the children grew older the needs changed, and mothers wanted particularly to know how to cope with the sexual development and sexual needs of their adult children, and again such advice was seldom available. Community nurses, who had had no contact with the Surrey mothers, would seem to be well placed to provide such information, or at least to offer access to appropriate information (Craft & Craft 1982; Maksym 1990).

Monetary allowances were very welcome but their allocation seemed capricious. As Shepperdson (1992) also notes, the more severely disabled children and young people did, on the whole, get the larger allowances but there were puzzling anomalies and contradictions. Whether a mother got an allowance often seemed to depend on her willingness to make a fuss, and on her persistence in doing so. Sheer luck also seemed, on occasions, to play a significant part in determining whether a mother found out about a particular fund, or whether the person assessing the child for an allowance was more or less sympathetic. While this works to the benefit of a determined mother who will not be put off, there are others who have at least equal needs but who lose out. There is a need for much better, and much more immediate, information on the allowances to which families are entitled; for clearer guidelines for those making assessments to enable them to be realistic about the difficulties faced by mothers of children with learning disabilities in general, and with Down's syndrome in particular; and for assessments that are at least as generous they have been in the past.

Parents have a number of implicit requirements of services and service providers. Firstly, they look for the service to give them a measure of relief – that is, the service should function, and continue to function, to the benefit of the parents. Secondly, families should be able to become aware of the service; the families should actively be made aware of its existence, and not left to find out about it by themselves or by chance. Thirdly, those providing the service should relate positively both to the disabled person and to the families, to let them see that they are respected as human beings and are not belittled because they are or have a family member who is disabled. Fourthly, service providers should recognise the individuality and variability of disabled people and their families, that they have the right to choose what and what not to accept, and that a service which seems to the providers to be precisely the right one may not be what this person or family wants. Byrne *et al.* (1988) also discuss the 'four criteria' by which mothers evaluate services from professionals; the first three are similar in content to those discussed above, their fourth, the effectiveness with which the professionals liaise with other agencies, although clearly of importance, was less evident in the Surrey group. Only the first has financial implications: the remainder require better training, better rationalisation of information resources, and a more sensitive approach to families on the part of some individuals in most of the professions.

NINE

Summary and conclusions

The developmental study

Like other groups of children with Down's syndrome, those in Surrey had relatively high scores on developmental tests in the first few months, the scores decreasing rapidly in early infancy and, in this group, more slowly after the age of 10 months. The decline continued to 11 years, so the rise at the age of 21 was the more unexpected. A substantial rise in IQ, in a similarly aged group of adults, has been shown elsewhere (Berry *et al.* 1984), although it is not clear how far this may have been due to the remedial programme in which the group was involved. Nevertheless, the downward curve of scores, seen in numerous studies in early childhood, may not inevitably continue. It has long been accepted that people with Down's syndrome continue to be able to learn and to develop skills well after the school-leaving age; it may be that, in the course of the learning that occurs in childhood and adolescence, they also acquire techniques, strategies and insights that can be applied to performance on psychological tests. In non-disabled populations, such an increase in skill at older ages occurs more commonly in relation to verbal than to non-verbal material. Given their relative difficulties with verbal material this might not be expected to hold good for people with Down's syndrome and indeed the opposite trend was seen in both the studies discussed: in the Surrey study the gain was seen on a non-verbal test (the Leiter scale) following one with some verbal content (the Merril–Palmer scale), and in the study by Berry *et al.* (1984) the gain on a non-verbal test (Raven's Matrices) was substantially greater than that on a verbal test (Peabody Picture Vocabulary Test). If future researchers seek for increases in scores on intelligence tests in adults with Down's syndrome, it seems likely that they will be found on non-verbal rather than on verbal tests. This would be consistent with the well-recognised finding that people with Down's syndrome have strengths in the visual rather than the auditory or vocal areas, but any such increase would, in supporting the findings already discussed, throw new light on the patterns of development in people with Down's syndrome.

As we move from a discussion of the data from the aggregated group to those of individuals within it, one of the most striking features of the study is the wide variation in ability shown by people with Down's syndrome. Although recognising that IQ scores do not have the same meaning at the extremities as they have over the middle part of the range, the range of scores in the Surrey group, of about 60 points, is of the same order as for the majority of the more to the less able in the normal population (IQs 70–130). Certainly, the difference experienced in a social encounter with one of the most able young people with Down's syndrome, and with one of the most severely disabled, is at least as great as that experienced in a school when encountering first a potential university candidate and then a member of a remedial class. This wide range of ability in people with Down's syndrome has been documented but little remarked on by researchers, and does not seem yet to have been fully appreciated by the general public.

Given this wide range of ability, it remains true that, despite relatively high correlations between IQs at different ages, attempts to predict the later IQ of any individual cannot be guaranteed to be successful. The position of most members of the cohort in relation to the rest remained fairly stable but for some there were large changes of scores from one age to another. These changes could go either way: on the one hand, the ability levels of a small number of those with high scores in infancy declined very sharply, while on the other those of a few improved, although more modestly. It should be noted that these phenomena, of large alterations in ability level over time, concerned a minority of those in the Surrey survey, fewer than 10% of the original sample. They have not been reported from other studies and need to be replicated if they are to be of real significance.

Where the development of self-help skills was concerned, overall the children with Down's syndrome acquired these in the same order as did the non-disabled children, but more slowly, and in some cases incompletely. Most skills were developed by age 11, after which further development, although still possible, was less often seen, and even as young adults nearly two-thirds were not able to look after their own self-care entirely. How far the young people will be able, in their twenties, to make up their skill deficiencies can be ascertained only by further research, but considering the data supplied by other studies (Holmes 1988; Shepperdson 1992) it seems virtually certain that some, at least, will continue to be significantly dependent. Inevitably this will place limits on the extent to which these young people will be able to lead independent lives in the community, and augers continued burdens of responsibility for their parents and carers.

A major finding, in both this and other studies (Ross 1971; Holmes 1988, p. 191; Turner *et al.* 1991) has been of the importance of IQ, the relationship to skill learning being similar to that relating to academic subjects (Carr 1988a). Both kinds of skill were more easily acquired by able than by less able children with Down's syndrome, although other factors, such as the opportunities and encouragement provided, were seen in individual cases to have been important. IQ is not, as has been claimed, 'probably one of the most trivial pieces of information to be ascertained' (Buddenhagen 1967, cited by Mittler 1973), but impacts significantly on a wide range of life domains of people with Down's syndrome and can provide useful pointers as to what should be expected of them. This may be especially valuable where an individual is found to be achieving less than he or she should be capable of, and may stimulate more efforts to help him or her to go further.

Behaviour

In the study of behaviour and its management three main points emerged. Firstly, there was a tendency for some personality and behaviour patterns to persist over time. Secondly, another tendency was seen for behaviours to improve; for the young people to be seen as easier to live with as they grew older. Thirdly, manifestations of behaviour were apparently independent of the management strategies that had been adopted earlier by the parents. These findings were not wholly expected, and particularly unexpected was the last, that the disciplinary approaches adopted by the parents could not be shown to have had any significant effect, for good or ill, on the behaviour of the young people. This finding could be said to have been particularly unwelcome: one of the functions that the present, longitudinal, study was expected to serve was that of providing pointers to the most effective ways of handling the young child with Down's syndrome, ways that would help him or her to grow up into a happy, well-adjusted individual who would be accepted and at home in social settings. Many mothers expressed uncertainty as to how they should deal with their children, whether the methods they had used with their other children would be appropriate or not, and many wished they could have had some expert advice on this. The hope that such advice would be forthcoming as a result of the findings of the present study has been largely unrealised. Our data, based on the analysis of the ways that the mothers reported themselves as dealing with their children, cannot be translated into much in the way of confident recommendations on the topic. Whether other, more sophisticated, disciplinary methods would have been more productive cannot be determined here. Only two mothers, both with very difficult 11 year old boys, had received some psychological advice, based on behavioural principles, on handling their sons, one mother remarking at 21 'It was the making of me'. However, these methods still await long-term validation, while it is extremely doubtful that they would be accepted on a large scale by families in the absence of particularly difficult behaviours in the child. So what can be offered to parents is a certain amount of reassurance, and some negative guidance (not 'Do this' but 'Don't do that'). Since it is not uncommon to find parents facing the teenage and adult years with apprehension ('what's it going to be like when he's bigger?'), it might be encouraging for them to know that this apprehension is, on the whole, unfounded. Most difficulties were not likely to be exacerbated as the children grew older; most of the young people were felt to be easier as adults than they had been as children, and this seemed to be due partly to the diminishing of some problem behaviours, and partly to gains in self-help ('he can do so much more for himself now'). Some parental anxieties could be allayed.

Where child rearing advice is concerned, there is little to suggest that any particular approach has anything to recommend it over another; nevertheless it can be said that physical punishment has not been shown to result in improvement in behaviour. On the contrary, its use on a regular basis and as the main form of discipline was followed by worse levels of behaviour in the Nottingham study, and the trends in the present and the Manchester studies were to some extent consistent with this.

This last finding, although negative, could be instructive. Many mothers who use smacking in disciplining their learning-disabled children say they do so because 'it's the only thing he understands'. The association between a short, sharp slap and here-and-now deterrence seems clear, but if the mothers are concerned, as many were, not only with the here-and-now but also with the future, and if they became aware that, far from having a reformative effect, smacking appears to be linked with greater behavioural difficulties in the future, they would be more hesitant about using it. As one mother said, apropos of the effect of smacking on her 4 year old with Down's syndrome, 'It stops him at the time but it doesn't really alter his behaviour'. This mother recognised that smacking was ineffective but had found it difficult to come up with anything better. She might have been helped to look more carefully at his behaviour, at the circumstances of and spin-offs from it; and then helped to ensure that the consequences of his 'good' behaviours were more to his liking than were those of his 'bad' ones. These strategies, of functional analysis and reinforcement, have much to commend them and seem likely to be more useful than simple smacking, but we are not, at present, in a position to know whether they would perform any better long-term than the other disciplinary methods that have come under research scrutiny.

Finally, there are indications that the atmosphere in the home, the warmth of the mother's relationship with and attitude to the child (perhaps also the father's), what Caldwell (1964) describes as the 'interpersonal context' of child rearing, may have some influence on the child's later adjustment. If this is so, then as well as trying to help parents of difficult children to develop more effective ways of handling them in the short-term, we should perhaps also be looking for ways to enable them to see and enjoy the positive aspects of their children's personalities and behaviours. In the long-term, this might pay dividends.

Living and life styles

When the subjects of this study were babies some mothers were given pessimistic prognostications about them – 'We thought she was always going to be a vegetable'; 'I thought he would always be chesty and snuffly' (Carr 1975). So when as 4 year olds they were seen as similar to the controls in their health, it seemed possible that, relieved to find them less fragile than they had feared, the mothers overestimated their robustness. However, views of their health have altered little over the years and most of the children and young people have experienced reasonably good health. Where there have been differences from the controls these were usually to the disadvantage of those with Down's syndrome – more had died, illnesses tended to be more serious, and vision, hearing and weight problems tended to be more prevalent. The exception was in the level of serious accidents, which, in contrast with the findings of Turner *et al.* (1990), were much less common in the Down's syndrome than in the control children. As Turner *et al.* (1990) also showed, a small number were identified who had multiple and serious health problems; these problems were associated in Turner *et al.*'s study with behaviour disorders, while in the present study there was a trend towards association with lower ability levels. Advances in medical care, which have already transformed the lives of some, may be expected to provide still more improvement in the well-being of people with Down's syndrome in the future; meantime the families of these individuals are likely to need more support to help them to cope not only with the problems of health but also with the difficulties associated with poor health.

If the cohort were doing better on health factors than had been anticipated, the same could not be said of their independence and social lives, which were noticeably more restricted than were those of the controls. Even as adults, two-thirds or more were never left in the house alone for as much as a few hours, or allowed to go outside the immediate neighbourhood; few took part in community events, and very few indeed were in or likely to gain employment. Fewer of those with Down's syndrome had friends; those friends they had they saw less of, and they were less likely to go out and about with them. Although many of the young people with Down's syndrome wished for relationships with the opposite sex, such relationships, which were the norm for the controls, for them were in the main discounted and discouraged. To some extent these differences could be accounted for by the degree of learning disability; as might be expected, those with more severe disabilities, and especially those with very severe and profound disabilities, were much less likely to have relationships and engage in activities that were run-of-the-mill for their non-disabled contemporaries. There were, however, many examples of individuals who did not take part in these activities who were quite as capable as others who did. Sometimes it seemed that the environment was responsible, sometimes the personality or behaviour patterns of the young person, but in a few cases it seemed that the factor holding the young person back was the parent's anxiety and disbelief in the competence and probable safety of their child. The feeling of parents, that it is they, above all, who care most deeply about the safety and well-being of their offspring, and who could never forgive themselves if, due to their negligence, anything untoward happened to him or her, must be respected. Nevertheless, some perhaps need to be encouraged to allow their sons and daughters to become more venturesome; they might be helped to do so if the transitions to greater independence were designed to take place gradually, and were accompanied by gradually diminishing safety precautions.

The effect on the families

In the first phase of the study, up to 4 years old, one of the most striking findings was that the difficulties the families experienced were not as numerous or severe as had been expected. The Down's syndrome babies were more difficult to feed, and when they became toddlers they were behind the controls in their skills, had more health problems, and were naughtier at a time when the controls had become more amenable. The mothers were more restricted in their outings, but in many respects – in the health of the mothers, helpfulness of fathers, family holidays, the manageability of the children, and the chores they entailed – there was little difference between the groups. None of the differences identified, with the exception of feeding, was thought by the mothers to constitute a serious problem. More cogent was the dread that many families felt of the future. These feelings seemed eminently reasonable, and with suitable caution it was pointed out that the rather rosy picture portrayed of the families 'applies, so far as we know, only until the children are 4 years old, and it is quite possible that as they get older and as the divergence between the normal child and the child with Down's syndrome becomes yet more marked, the difficulties may become greater' (Carr 1975, p. 131). With the present phases of the study we have moved well beyond that time, the divergence between the two groups has certainly become more marked; to the point where in most skill areas there was virtually no overlap between them. However, where the effect of the Down's syndrome person on family life is considered, differences were less pronounced. This was especially true in regard to the effect on the sibs, an area of great concern to almost all parents, and one which they confronted almost as soon as the diagnosis of the baby was made. In common with most other up-to-date studies, few serious adverse effects on the sibs have been found. Relationships between them were as good as in any other family (rather better in some respects); sibs were not discouraged from having other friends, nor from bringing these friends into the home; no differences could be seen in the health or behaviour of the sibs in the two groups, neither concurrently nor longitudinally. Undoubtedly some sibs may be found who are distressed by the presence of a disabled brother or sister but for the great majority this is not the case.

Looking at the effect on the mothers, many positive features emerged. Although about half felt at some point that they had been made lonely by having a disabled child, this persisted in only a tiny minority and was stoutly rebutted by many. In common with most other studies of families with a Down's syndrome child, there was, in the present one, no evidence of a higher rate of marital discord, or of divorce. Despite going out less, mothers in the Down's syndrome group were no less content with the degree to which they went out. In other areas, however, the mothers in the Down's syndrome group were disadvantaged. They were severely hampered in their freedom to go out to work, this becoming increasingly difficult as the individual with Down's syndrome grew to adulthood, and was in most cases directly attributable to the responsibility the mother had for him or her. The finding in the 4 year phase of greater restriction on the mothers' social lives was supported, although to a lesser extent, as the children grew older, but most mothers seemed to adapt to their situation without resentment. Mothers are good at making the best of things, and those who find this more difficult may be those who are more stressed and depressed. Byrne *et al.* (1988) make the point that families of children with behaviour disorders were more likely to *feel* restricted, although in fact they went out as much as did families whose children did not have such difficult behaviours, and suggest that what these families need is not so much more breaks from their children as interventions that would 'help them to feel more positive about their child's behaviour and more capable of dealing with it and understanding it'. Practical help for families should not be forgotten; Beresford (1993) shows that financial help can ease some burdens, and Byrne *et al.* (1988) single out the need for parents of children with serious medical conditions to have access to babysitters who have the expertise that will allow the parents to feel free to go out. In addition, it cannot be said too strongly that, if the old-style programmes of generalised stimulation for infants with Down's syndrome are not now seen as appropriate, there is a clear need for families, and especially the parents, to be provided with sympathetic support, access to information, and, where necessary, other help such as guidance on child-rearing and management. There may too be some whose personalities make them less able to deal with all the extra problems of a disabled child. These parents might benefit, as Byrne *et al.* (1988, p. 141) suggest, from a dual approach that teaches them strategies for handling the child, and, on a more personal level, more positive ways of viewing and valuing him or her.

In the late 1960s, there was much discussion of 'the handicapped family' (Goldie 1966), which was seen as the near-inevitable result of the birth of a disabled child, and this view was supported by gloomy first-hand accounts from distressed parents (Hannam 1980). Marriages were expected to disintegrate under the strain, the evidence for this resting largely on one study of families of children severely physically disabled by spina bifida (Tew, Payne & Laurence 1974). Follow-up of these same families some nine years later found no difference in marital harmony between the groups (Evans, Tew & Laurence 1986), but the 1974 study continues to be cited as evidence of the vulnerability of marriage in families containing a learning-disabled child. More recently, and especially through the application of epidemiological research methods, involving the study of populations and not just that of disaffected and articulate volunteers, the picture has changed. The variability of the families, of their situations, the problems and stresses that they face, and the strengths and resources they have, are recognised and documented. Byrne *et al.* (1988, p. 135) speak of 'an overwhelming impression of family normality, variety and strength'. Certainly, a number of families have problems and some are under severe strain, and one of the major needs for the future is to pursue the identification of those families and to ensure they get the help they need. But for others, perhaps the majority, the predominant impression they give is of resilience and the ability to cope with their situation. The need now is for this to be more widely known and acknowledged; for some professionals to put aside their armchair convictions about the burdens that they intuitively know are carried by families with a disabled member, and to give credence to findings, from properly conducted research, based on the views of the parents themselves.

Such a parent-orientated perspective would be consistent with the result of shifts that have taken place in the views of service-deliverers on the most appropriate ways of helping families. These have gone from adherence to the early, 'professional-centred' models, in which professionals were the 'experts', who made decisions for families, who were seen as unable to cope on their own; to the 'family-allied' models in which families carried out the instructions of a professional; through to the more recently developed 'family-centred' model in which families 'determine all aspects of service delivery and resource provision', and professionals are there to support them and to 'promote family decision-making, capabilities and competencies' (Dunst *et al.* 1991). The authors carried out a survey of policy-makers and practitioners, which showed 'a movement toward adoption of family-centered early intervention policies and practices'; while the survey was conducted in the USA the same tendencies can be seen also in this country, and may similarly be expected to result in better outcomes for the families.

The role of services

Almost all reviews of services for people with disabilities find them to be inadequate and failing to meet identified needs: almost all finish with a list of improvements that need to be made. The review given in Chapter 8 is no exception, yet it must be said that, flawed as they are, the services in existence do a great deal to ease the lot of the families. Prominent among these are the schools, which in the earliest years not only provide the much-wanted education for the children but also give the mothers some respite from the day-long task of caring. Day centres play a similar role when the children become adults but are seen to have more drawbacks to them than was the case for the schools. This may be partly because of the ever-widening gap between the lives of the young people with Down's syndrome and their non-disabled peers; the difference between them, in the types of activity engaged in and the prospects that lie before them, being even clearer than it was during their school days. A number of recommendations have been made for: an increase in the number and variety of courses offered by the centres, better training for centre staff to enable them to pursue more vigorously employment possibilities for their clients (Holmes 1988, pp. 431–2); a structure to the centre day that resembles that of a work environment rather than a school – 'Down's adults like to think of themselves as going out to work like the rest of the family' (Lane 1985, p. 399); and, perhaps implicit in the last but needing special emphasis, longer and more flexible hours, which would enable those mothers who wanted to do so to take up employment that was realistically related to their wishes and talents.

Medical services were much appreciated, especially, it seemed, where hospital doctors were concerned, when they had a particular function to perform and hospital appointments were not a matter of routine, which in the early years mothers found irksome and pointless. Family doctors play a crucial role as the first people to whom parents of new babies and toddlers turn; even if they do not think of themselves as having expertise in the area of Down's syndrome, they can provide vital support to parents if they are willing to give the child with Down's syndrome as much attention as they would give to any other child – not a great deal to ask. Doctors cannot cure Down's syndrome nor do the parents expect them to. Nevertheless, they can do much to alleviate the condition, especially as the individual grows older, not only by attending to the medical problems that arise but also in being alert to those that may otherwise go unnoticed, such as the onset of hearing or thyroid disorders; this will be to the benefit of the people with Down's syndrome and, indirectly, to their families.

Social workers can be an important link for families with a whole range of relief services, and can be of particular importance in informing them of the financial benefits to which they are entitled, and better still, in helping them to apply for and obtain them. Here again the human element plays a part, the friendship and interest offered by the social worker to both the child and the family being almost equally valued. This relationship cannot, however, be expected to flourish if the social worker is so overstretched that he or she does not have enough time to give the family, or is unreliable; still less if staff turnover is so rapid that the relationship cannot be established. The provision of respite and short-term care is seen, rightly, as offering parents and families breaks in the routine of day-to-day care. Nevertheless, parents are likely to reject such offers, no matter how much they themselves feel in need of them, unless they are convinced that the standard of care provided is such that they would be happy about the child's welfare. Until then, and especially while the child is young, even though it seems that it is then that the families' need of respite is greatest, many parents will prefer to forego the breaks they need and want.

Inevitably, some of the needs expressed by parents, and of the recommendations proposed to meet these needs, have considerable resource implications, which have little likelihood of being provided. Other needs could be met more economically, and it may be worth while reiterating these: the need for all professionals to treat people with Down's syndrome, and their families, with as much respect as is due to any human being; to extend this respect to their individuality, to make no assumptions about their situation and wishes but to listen to what they have to say; and for information on all topics relevant to them to be available and accessible. These needs could be met partly by better (but not greatly extended) professional training, and also by more involvement with the media, especially television. Much of the more accepting attitude on the part of the public, which families have acknowledged, is already attributed to the realistic but sympathetic depiction on our screens of people with Down's syndrome. The process should be carried further to increase the awareness of public and professionals alike of the real lives of people with Down's syndrome and of their families.

Looking to the future

Many changes have taken place since the time when the present cohort was born. Life expectancy for people with Down's syndrome has increased, advances in pharmacology have changed the outlook for those subject to infections and in surgical techniques for those with heart problems. Babies whose families do not feel able to bring them up themselves are no longer placed in institutions, and indeed are in demand for adoption. The long-term future for an infant born with Down's syndrome today is envisaged as in the community and not, as the Surrey mothers anticipated with horror, in the back ward of a 'subnormality' hospital. Looking ahead from the vantage point of these changes, what further developments may we expect over the next few decades? Developments there are certain to be, and they can be envisaged as occurring in the medical, the psycho-educational, and the socio-ecological fields.

The medical advances that have already taken place are likely to be followed by further advances in the same significant areas, with greater sophistication of surgical techniques and new and more effective antibiotic treatments. Similarly, more effective ways of treating thyroid and hearing problems may be developed. Much research is currently underway into Alzheimer's disease, and important discoveries are being made regarding genetic aspects of the disease (Hodes 1994), which may lead to greater understanding, possibly even to some amelioration, of the disease process. Any or all of these advances would improve the health of people with Down's syndrome and lead to further increases in their lifespan.

Moving from the medical to the psycho-educational field, the first point to note is the change that has already occurred in some areas. At the conclusion of the report on the first phase of the study, high hopes were held for the benefits for people with Down's syndrome that were expected from early intervention projects: 'All [early intervention studies] have shown, despite certain methodological drawbacks, considerable developmental advantage in the children whose mothers were involved over those whose mothers were not involved in the early intervention programmes' (Carr 1975, pp. 134–5). The passage goes on to outline how such a programme would run, and the advantages likely to ensue for both child and mother.

Since then, with the passing of almost two decades in which these pro-grammes have been conducted and evaluated, the early hopes have not been realised, and firm research evidence of long-term benefits to the children from the programmes, especially in cognitive domains, is lacking (Cunningham 1987; Gibson 1991). Some permanent effects have been seen: children who have been involved in the programmes had fewer major health problems, were more likely to be reported by their mothers as having hearing and visual difficulties, and were more likely to have attended a mixed or mainstream pre-school facility; also, their mothers were more likely to be in work and to be willing to leave the child unsupervised for longer periods (Cunningham 1987). As Cunningham (1987) remarks, these indicate greater self-confidence on the part of the intervention mothers, and their greater awareness and willingness to seek help. These are valuable effects, but they do not suggest a significant positive effect on the children themselves. If, now, mothers of new babies were invited to join an early intervention programme and were told what were likely to be the effects of it – predominantly on their own self-confidence and awareness – it seems doubtful that many would take up the offer, especially when the not-inconsiderable strains of such programmes on the family are taken into account (Mittler 1979; Turnbull & Turnbull 1982).

It is now accepted in many quarters that generalised, non-specific pro-grammes of coaching and stimulation of Down's syndrome infants do not confer the advantages that were expected from them (Cunningham 1987; Gibson & Harris 1988; Wishart 1991). Attention is turning, then, to the question of whether there are specific difficulties experienced by people with Down's syndrome that might be addressed and ameliorated. Gibson (1978) provides an extensive review of the literature on the particular characteristics of people with Down's syndrome, which, briefly summar-ised, shows relative strength in visual-motor skills and rote memory, and relatively poor performance with audio-vocal material, in tactile-shape rec-ognition, motor speed, language, and number skills. Later writers have sup-ported many of these findings, e.g. those on language (Kernan 1990). In a more recent publication Gibson (1991, pp. 80–1) identifies a wide range of strengths and weaknesses of people with Down's syndrome, too numerous to reproduce in full here, but including strengths in gestural communi-cation, rote memory and memory for form, and weaknesses in attention, persistence and judgement, comprehension, and reasoning. Gibson (1991) proposes that the strengths should be 'intensely exploited' in the reme-diation of the weaknesses.

A series of studies from Edinburgh has isolated a number of ways in which the learning processes of infants with Down's syndrome differ from those of non-disabled infants. Examples include: 'a narrow range of engagement', that is an avoidance of tasks that were too difficult and also, interestingly, of those that were too easy; failure to consolidate skills, so that tasks that were passed on one occasion were failed or refused on another, and hence a failure to build on previously acquired skills; the avoidance of aversive demands by 'switching out' or by the use of social skills (catching and holding the experimenter's eye and refusing to attend to the task, or resorting to 'party tricks' such as clapping or blowing raspberries) these behaviours being abandoned if the difficulty level of the task was reduced to be within the infant's developmental range (Wishart 1986, 1988, 1990); passivity in the face of a task where a large measure of control of a reinforcing stimulus was possible, and acceptance of a much lower rate of freely available reinforcement (Wishart 1990); and response to errorless learning and trial-and-error approaches that differed from that of non-disabled infants (Duffy & Wishart 1987). These discoveries point to particular areas of difficulty, not found in the non-disabled infant, which if they could be remediated (and this could certainly be attempted) should open up the way forward for these young children in ways that, until now, have not been undertaken.

Cunningham (1987) also believes that intervention must take a path different from that followed hitherto, suggesting that intervention should 'encompass individual differences and aim at specific targets'. He feels that in the early years social-interactive models may be more productive than sensory-motor training but that training in independent functioning should continue; he emphasises the need for support and counselling to be provided for parents.

There are, therefore, potentially valuable approaches by which the learning and skills of the child with Down's syndrome might be enhanced, and they generate optimism for the future. This optimism is tempered, somewhat, by awareness of the obstacles that lie between the research discoveries described above and their implementation in educational regimes for children with Down's syndrome. To date, so far as this author is aware, the research remains just that, and there is no indication that any of the findings are being incorporated into classroom routines. Indeed, it is not clear just how this should be done. One of the strong points of the early intervention programmes was that it was relatively obvious what teaching they involved. Based, as they were, on normal child development, a graded succession of skills could be targeted and each could be focused on in turn in ways that made sense to both teachers and parents. The situation is much less clear in regard to the more recent research findings, and very little in the way of programmes has been drawn up. Given that this is done, it will then be necessary for the programmes to be put into practice and their long-term effectiveness evaluated. There is, then, still a long way to go before it will be possible to conclude that we have reliable ways of enhancing the abilities of children with Down's syndrome, but there are grounds for not only hoping but expecting that this will come about.

Lastly, we may look to the field of social and community involvement for indications of the progress to be made in the position held by people with Down's syndrome in society. Increasingly they live in the community but their participation in its life has been, with some rare exceptions, very limited. Very few are in employment, their activities tend to be in segregated rather than ordinary facilities, their friends are others with learning disabilities, and, like people with other forms of learning disabilities, they experience loneliness and social isolation (Landesman-Dwyer 1981; Saxby *et al.* 1986, Ward 1988). Efforts are being made world-wide to address these problems, from providing training in the skills needed for community living (Lindsay *et al.* 1988) to increasing access to normal work environments (Nilsson 1988), and to setting up volunteer friendship schemes (Prenderville 1988; Roberts *et al.* 1988). We may expect, in the future, to see many more opportunities for people with Down's syndrome, and those with other learning disabilities, to participate in ordinary community activities. In so doing, we may need to keep in mind the primary necessity, that of enabling the people concerned to make their own choices. The motivation behind many of the initiatives detailed above has rested on theories of normalisation, with the ideal that people with learning disabilities should not only live but also fully participate in normal communities and normal life. These aims and ideas now govern the thinking of many, perhaps the majority, of those working in the field of learning disability in this, and most developed countries, and are humanitarian in their intent. It is to be hoped that they will not lead to the disregard of the signals that may come from the people with learning disabilities themselves. Although studies have found that many learning-disabled people relish the chance to take part in normal activities, this may not be the choice for some, or for some in some circumstances. Neumayer, Smith & Lundegren (1993) found that people with Down's syndrome, offered the choice of engaging in leisure activities with non-disabled people or with others with Down's syndrome, chose significantly more often to go with others with Down's syndrome. There may have been a variety of reasons for this choice, and one of the first questions to be asked is, was it an informed choice? Especially where a choice is made *not* to participate in an activity, this may be, at least in part, because the person has no experience of it and does not in fact know what it is that he or she is rejecting. We have then to ensure that opportunities are not denied to people with Down's syndrome through ignorance; but equally we should not be so ruled by adherence to ideological principles that we ride rough shod over the wishes of the people concerned. 'The belief that *all* people with mental retardation will have an improved quality of life through compulsory integration into all aspects of society at all times . . . is questionable' (Neumayer *et al.* 1993). Landesman-Dwyer (1981) recommends that we assess (and presumably promote) the quality of life as much as possible 'from the viewpoint of individual clients – their personal preferences, needs, and capabilities – rather than from our own perspective (e.g. "Would *I* like to live here?")'. With that goal in mind, it may be that real advances can be made in building a better life for people with Down's syndrome.

References

* Original references not seen.

Abramovitch, R., Stanhope, L., Pepler, D. & Corter, C. (1987). The influence of Down's syndrome on sibling interaction. *Journal of Child Psychology and Psychiatry*, **28**, 865–879.

Anderson, E.M. & Clarke, L. (1982). *Disability in adolescence*. London: Methuen.

Baird, P.A. & Sadovnik, A.D. (1988). Life expectancy in Down syndrome adults. *Lancet*, **ii**, 1354–1356.

Baldwin, S.M. (1985). *The costs of caring: families with a disabled child*. London: Routledge & Kegan Paul.

Barden, H.S. (1985). Dentition and other aspects of growth and development. In *Current approaches to Down's syndrome*, ed. D. Lane & B. Stratford, pp. 71–84. London & New York: Holt, Rinehart & Winston.

Baron, J. (1972). Temperament profile of children with Down's syndrome. *Development Medicine and Child Development*, **14**, 640–643.

Bayley, N. (1969). *Manual for the Bayley Scales on infant development*. New York: Psychological Corporation.

Bayley, N., Rhodes, L. & Gooch, B. (1966). A comparison of the development of institutionalized and home-reared mongoloids. *California Mental Health Research Digest*, **4**, 104–105.

Bell, A.J. & Bhate, M.S. (1992). Prevalence of overweight and obesity in Down's syndrome and other mentally handicapped adults living in the community. *Journal of Intellectual Disability Research*, **36**, 359–364.

Bennett, F.C., Sells, C.J. & Brand, C. (1979). Influences on measured intelligence in Down's syndrome. *American Journal of Diseases in Childhood*, **50**, 383–386.

Beresford, B.A. (1993). Easing the strain: assessing the impact of a Family Fund grant on mothers caring for a severely disabled child. *Child: Care, Health and Development*, **19**, 369–378.

Berger, J. & Cunningham, C. (1983). Early social interaction between infants with Down's syndrome and their parents. *Health Visitor*, **56**, 58–60.

Berry, P., Groenweg, G., Gibson, D. & Brown, R.I. (1984). Mental development of adults with Down syndrome. *American Journal of Mental Deficiency*, **89**, 252–256.

Berry, P., Gunn, P., Andrews, R. & Price, C. (1981). Characteristics of Down syndrome infants and their families. *Australian Paediatric Journal*, **17**, 40–43.

Bilovsky, D. & Share, J. (1965). The ITPA and Down's syndrome: an exploratory study. *American Journal of Mental Deficiency*, **70**, 78–82.

Blacketer-Simmonds, D.A. (1953). An investigation into the supposed difference existing between mongols and other mentally defective subjects with regard to certain psychological traits. *Journal of Mental Science*, **99**, 702–719.

Bose, R. (1991). The effect of a family support scheme on maternal mental health of mothers caring for children with mental handicaps. *Research, Policy and Planning*, **9**, 2–7.

Boyce, G.C. & Barnett, W.S. (1993). Siblings of persons with mental retardation: a historical perspective and recent findings. In *The effects of mental retardation, disability and illness*, ed. Z. Stoneman & P.W. Berman, pp. 145–184. Baltimore: P.H. Brookes.

Boyce, G.C., Barnett, W.S. & Miller, B.C. (1991). Time use and attitudes among siblings: a comparison in families of children with and without Down syndrome. Poster presented at the Biennial Meeting of the Society for Research in Child Development, Seattle, WA, USA.

Bradshaw, J.R. (1980). *The Family Fund*. London: Routledge & Kegan Paul.

Bradshaw, J.R. (1982). *Evaluating the Malaise Inventory: a comparison of measures of stress*. Report to DHSS, 96, 3/82, MH/JB.

Brimblecombe, F.S.W. (1979). A new approach to the care of handicapped children. *Journal of the Royal College of Physicians of London*, **13**, 231–236.

*Bristol, M., Gallagher, J. & Schopler, E. (1987). Mothers and fathers of young developmentally disabled and nondisabled boys: adaptation and spousal support. *Developmental Psychology*, **24**, 441–451.

British Medical Journal (1977). Diagnostic amniocentesis in early pregnancy. Annotation, **1**, 1430–1431.

*Brothwell, D.R. (1960). *Annals of Human Genetics*, **24**, 141.

Buckley, S. (1985). Attaining basic educational skills: reading, writing and number. In *Current Approaches to Down's syndrome*, ed. D. Lane & B. Stratford, pp. 315–343. London & New York: Holt, Rinehart & Winston.

Buckley, S. & Sacks, B. (1987). *The adolescent with Down's syndrome*. Portsmouth Polytechnic.

Buddenhagen, R.G. (1967). Towards a better understanding. *Mental Retardation*, **5**, 40–41.

Burden, R.L. (1980). Measuring the effects of stress on mothers of handicapped infants: must depression always follow? *Child: Care, Health and Development*, **6**, 165–171.

Burton, L. (1975). *The family life of sick children*. London: Routledge & Kegan Paul.

Butterfield, E.C. (1961). A provocative case of over-achievement by a mongoloid. *American Journal of Mental Deficiency*, **66**, 444–448.

Byrne, E.A., Cunningham, C.C. & Sloper, P. (1988). *Families and their children with Down's syndrome*. London: Routledge.

Caldwell, B.M. (1964). The effects of infant care. In *Review of child development research*, vol. 1, ed. M.L. Hoffman & L.W. Hoffman, pp. 21–87. New York: Russell Sage Foundation.

Carr, J. (1970). Mongolism: telling the parents. *Journal of Mental Deficiency Research*, **14**, 213–221.

Carr, J. (1975). *Young children with Down's syndrome.* London: Butterworths.

Carr, J. (1985). The development of intelligence. In *Current approaches to Down's syndrome,* ed. D. Lane & B. Stratford, pp. 167–186. London & New York: Holt, Rinehart & Winston.

Carr, J. (1988). Six weeks to twenty-one years old: a longitudinal study of children with Down's syndrome and their families. *Journal of Child Psychology & Psychiatry,* **29,** 407–431.

Carr, J. (1992a). Assets and deficits in the behaviour of people with Down's syndrome – a longitudinal study. In *Vulnerability and resilience in human development,* ed. B. Tizard & V. Varma, pp. 57–71. London: Jessica Kingsley Publishers.

Carr, J. (1992b). Longitudinal research in Down's syndrome. In *International review of research in mental retardation,* ed. N.W. Bray, vol. 18, pp. 197–223. San Diego: Academic Press.

Carr, J. & Hewett, S. (1982). Children with Down's syndrome growing up. *Association of Child Psychology and Psychiatry News,* **4,** 10–13.

Carr, J., Pearson, A. & Halliwell, M. (1983). *The GLC Spina Bifida survey: Follow-up at 11 and 12 years.* London: GLC Research and Statistics Branch.

Chess, S. & Thomas, A. (1984). *Origins and evolution of behavior disorders: from infancy to adult life.* New York: Brunner-Mazel.

Chess, S., Thomas, A. & Birch, H.G. (1966). Distortions in developmental reporting made by parents of behaviorally disturbed children. *Journal of the American Academy of Child Psychiatry,* **858,** 226–234.

Clarke, A.D.B. & Clarke, A.M. (1984). Constancy and change in the growth of human characteristics. *Journal of Child Psychology and Psychiatry,* **25,** 191–210.

Clements, P.R., Bates, M.V. & Hafer, M. (1976). Variability within Down's syndrome (Trisomy-21): empirically observed sex differences in IQs. *Mental Retardation,* **14,** 30–31.

Collacott, R.A. (1992). The effect of age and residential placement on adaptive behaviour of adults with Down's syndrome. *British Journal of Psychiatry,* **161,** 675–679.

Collacott, R.A. & Cooper, S.-A. (1992). Adaptive behaviour after depressive illness in Down's syndrome. *Journal of Nervous and Mental Disease,* **180,** 468–470.

Collacott, R.A., Cooper, S.-A. & McGrother, C. (1992). Differential rates of psychiatric disorders in adults with Down's syndrome compared with other mentally handicapped adults. *British Journal of Psychiatry,* **161,** 671–674.

*Collman, R.D. & Stoller, A. (1962). A survey of mongoloid births in Victoria, Australia, in 1942–1957. *American Journal of Public Health,* **52,** 813–829.

Cone, T. (1968). Is Down's syndrome a modern disease? *Lancet,* ii, 829.

Connolly, B., Morgan, S., Russell, F. & Richardson, B. (1980). Early intervention with Down's syndrome children: a follow-up report. *Physical Therapy,* **60,** 1405–1408.

Connolly, J.A. (1978). Intelligence levels of Down's syndrome children. *American Journal of Mental Deficiency,* **83,** 193–196.

Cook, E.H. & Leventhal, B.L. (1987). Down's syndrome and mania. *British Journal of Psychiatry,* **150,** 249–250.

Cooper, S.-A. & Collacott, R.A. (1991). Manic episodes in Down's syndrome: two case reports. *Journal of Nervous and Mental Disease,* 179, 635–636.

Corbett, J.A. (1973). Neuropsychiatric handicaps in children with severe mental retardation. Paper given at the Third Meeting of United Kingdom Paediatric Neurologists, Oxford.

Corbett, J.A. (1975). Aversion for the treatment of self-injurious behaviour. *Journal of Mental Deficiency Research,* 19, 79–95.

Cornwell, A.C. (1974). Development of language, abstraction and numerical concept formation in home-reared children with Down's syndrome (Mongolism). *American Journal of Mental Deficiency,* 74, 179–190.

Cornwell, A.C. & Birch, H.G. (1969). Psychological and social development in home-reared children with Down's syndrome (mongolism). *American Journal of Mental Deficiency,* 74, 341–350.

Cottrell, D.J. & Crisp, A.H. (1984). Anorexia nervosa in Down's syndrome – a case report. *British Journal of Psychiatry,* 145, 195–196.

Craft, M. & Craft, A. (1982). *Sex and the mentally handicapped.* 2nd edition. London: Royal College of Psychiatrists.

Cunningham, C.C. (1982). Psychological and educational aspects of handicap. In *Inborn errors of metabolism,* ed. F. Cockburn & R. Gitzelman, pp. 237–253. Lancaster: MTP Press.

Cunningham, C.C. (1987). Early intervention in Down's syndrome. In *Prevention of mental handicap: a world view* (RSM Services International Congress and Symposium Series No.112), ed. G. Hosking & G. Murphy, pp. 169–182. London: Royal Society of Medicine Services Ltd.

Cunningham, C. & McArthur, K. (1981). Hearing loss and treatment in young Down's syndrome children. *Child: Care, Health and Development,* 7, 357–374.

Cunningham, C.C., Morgan, P.A. & McGucken, R.B. (1984). Down's syndrome: is dissatisfaction with the diagnosis inevitable? *Developmental Medicine and Child Neurology,* 26, 33–39.

Cunningham, C. & Sloper, T. (1977). Parents of Down's syndrome babies: their early needs. *Child: Care, Health and Development,* 3, 325–347.

Cuskelly, M. & Gunn, P. (1993). Maternal reports of behavior of siblings of children with Down syndrome. *American Journal on Mental Retardation,* 97, 521–529.

*Dalton, A. & Crapper-McLachlan, D.R. (1984) Incidence of memory deterioration in ageing persons with Down's syndrome. In *Perspectives and progress in mental retardation,* vol. 2, ed. J.M. Berg, pp. 55–62. Baltimore, MD: University Park Press.

Dalton, A.J. & Wisniewski, H.M. (1990). Down's syndrome and the dementia of Alzheimer disease. *International Review of Psychiatry,* 2, 43–52.

Dameron, L.E. (1963). Development of intelligence of infants with mongolism. *Child Development,* 34, 733–738.

Demissie, A., Ayres, R.C. & Briggs, R. (1988). Old age in Down's syndrome. *Journal of the Royal Society of Medicine,* 81, 740.

Dicks-Mireaux, M.J. (1966). Development of intelligence in children with Down's syndrome: a preliminary report. *Journal of Mental Deficiency Research*, 10, 89–93.

Dicks-Mireaux, M.J. (1972). Mental development of infants with Down's syndrome. *American Journal of Mental Deficiency*, 77, 26–32.

Domino, G. (1965). Personality traits in institutionalized mongoloids. *American Journal of Mental Deficiency*, 69, 568–570.

Domino, G., Goldschmid, M. & Kaplan, M. (1964). Personality traits of institutionalized mongoloid girls. *American Journal of Mental Deficiency*, 68, 498–502.

Douglas, J.W.B., Lawson, A., Cooper, J.R. & Cooper, E. (1968). Family interaction and the activities of young children. *Journal of Child Psychology and Psychiatry*, 9, 157–171.

Down, J.L.H. (1866). Observations on an ethnic classification of idiots. *Clinical Lectures and Reports, London Hospital*, 3, 259–262.

*Duffen, L. (1976). Teaching reading to children with little or no language. *Remedial Education*, 11, 139.

Duffy, L. & Wishart, J. (1987). A comparison of two procedures for teaching discrimination skills to Down's syndrome and non-handicapped children. *British Journal of Educational Psychology*, 57, 265–278.

Dunn, L.M., Dunn, L.M., Whetton, C. & Pintilie, D. (1982). *The British Picture Vocabulary Scale*. Windsor: NFER-Nelson.

Dunsdon, M.I., Carter, C.O. & Huntley, R.M.C. (1960). Upper end of range of intelligence in mongolism. *Lancet*, i, 565–568.

Dunst, C.J., Johanson, C., Trivette, C.M. & Hamby, D. (1991). Family-oriented early intervention policies and practices: family centered or not? *Exceptional Children*, 58, 115–126.

Dupont, A., Vaeth, M. & Videbech, P. (1986). Mortality and life expectancy of Down's syndrome in Denmark. *Journal of Mental Deficiency Research*, 30, 111–120.

Ellis, A. & Beechley, R.M. (1950). A comparison of matched groups of mongoloid and non-mongoloid feeble-minded children. *American Journal of Mental Deficiency*, 54, 464–468.

Evans, O., Tew, B. & Laurence, K.M. (1986). The fathers of children with spina bifida. *Zeitschrift für Kinderchirurgie*, 41, 42–44.

Farber, B. (1959). Effects of a severely retarded child on family integration. *Monograph of the Society for Research into Child Development*, No. 71, vol. 24 No. 2.

Fenner, M.E., Hewitt, K.E. & Torpy, M. (1987). Down's syndrome: intellectual and behavioural functioning during adulthood. *Journal of Mental Deficiency Research*, 31, 241–246.

Ferguson, N. & Watt, J. (1980). The mothers of children with special educational needs. *Scottish Educational Review*, 12, 21–31.

Ferguson-Smith, M.A. (1983). Prenatal chromosome analysis and its impact on the birth incidence of chromosome disorders. *British Medical Bulletin*, 39, 355–364.

Fishler, K. & Koch, R. (1991). Mental development in Down syndrome mosaicism. *American Journal of Mental Deficiency,* **96,** 345–351.

Fowle, C.M. (1968). The effect of the severely retarded child on his family. *American Journal of Mental Deficiency,* **73,** 468–473.

Fowler, A.E. (1990). Language abilities in children with Down syndrome: evidence for a specific syntactic delay. In *Children with Down syndrome,* ed. D. Cicchetti & M. Beeghly, pp. 302–328. Cambridge: Cambridge University Press.

Fraser, F.C. & Sadovnik, A.D. (1976). Correlation of IQ in subjects with Down syndrome and their parents and sibs. *Journal of Mental Deficiency Research,* **20,** 179–182.

*Fraser, J. & Mitchell, A. (1876). Kalmuc idiocy: report of a case with autopsy with notes on 62 cases. *Journal of Mental Science* **22,** 161.

Friedrich, W.N. & Friedrich, W.L. (1981). Psychosocial assets of parents of handicapped and non-handicapped children. *American Journal of Mental Deficiency,* **85,** 551–553.

Friedrich, W.N., Wilturner, L.T. & Cohen, D.S. (1985). Coping resources and parenting mentally retarded children. *American Journal of Mental Deficiency,* **90,** 130–139.

Fryers, T. (1984). *The epidemiology of intellectual impairment.* London: Academic Press.

Gath, A. (1973). The school age siblings of mongol children. *British Journal of Psychiatry,* **123,** 161–167.

Gath, A. (1974). Sibling reactions to mental handicap: a comparison of the brothers and sisters of mongol children. *Journal of Child Psychology and Psychiatry,* **15,** 187–198.

Gath, A. (1985a). Down's syndrome in the first nine years. In *Longitudinal studies in child psychology and psychiatry,* ed. A.R. Nichol, pp. 203–219. Chichester: John Wiley & Sons Ltd.

Gath, A. (1985b). Parental reactions to loss and disappointment: the diagnosis of Down's syndrome. *Developmental Medicine and Child Neurology,* **27,** 392–400.

Gath, A. & Gumley, D. (1984). Down's syndrome and the family: follow-up of children first seen in infancy. *Developmental Medicine and Child Neurology,* **26,** 500–508.

Gath, A. & Gumley, D. (1986a). Behaviour problems in retarded children with special reference to Down's syndrome. *British Journal of Psychiatry,* **149,** 156–161.

Gath, A. & Gumley, D. (1986b). Family background of children with Down's syndrome and of children with a similar degree of mental retardation. *British Journal of Psychiatry,* **149,** 161–171.

Gath, A. & Gumley, D. (1987). Retarded children and their siblings. *Journal of Child Psychology and Psychiatry,* **28,** 715–730.

Gedye, A. (1990). Dietary increase in serotonin reduces self-injurious behaviour in a Down's syndrome adult. *Journal of Mental Deficiency Research,* **34,** 195–203.

Gibbs, M.V. & Thorpe, J.G. (1983). Personality stereotype of non-institutionalized Down syndrome children. *American Journal of Mental Deficiency,* **83,** 601–605.

Gibson, D. (1978). *Down's syndrome: the psychology of mongolism*. Cambridge: Cambridge University Press.

Gibson, D. (1991). Searching for a life-span psychobiology of Down syndrome: advancing educational and behavioural management strategies. *International Journal of Disability, Development and Education*, 38, 71–89.

Gibson, D. & Harris, A. (1988). Aggregated early intervention effects for Down's syndrome persons: patterning and longevity of benefits. *Journal of Mental Deficiency Research*, 32, 1–17.

Golden, W. & Pashayan, H.M. (1976). The effect of parental education on the eventual mental development of non-institutionalized children with Down syndrome. *Journal of Pediatrics*, 89, 403–407.

Goldie, L. (1966). The psychiatry of the handicapped family. *Developmental Medicine and Child Neurology*, 8, 456–462.

Goodman, N. & Tizard, J. (1962). The prevalence of imbecility and idiocy among children. *British Medical Journal*, 1, 216–219.

Gunn, P. & Berry, P. (1985). The temperament of Down's syndrome toddlers and their siblings. *Journal of Child Psychology and Psychiatry*, 26, 973–979.

Gunn, P., Berry, P. & Andrews, R.J. (1981). The temperament of Down's syndrome infants: a research note. *Journal of Child Psychology and Psychiatry*, 22, 189–194.

Gunn, P., Berry, P. & Andrews, R.J. (1983). The temperament of Down's syndrome toddlers: a research note. *Journal of Child Psychology and Psychiatry*, 24, 601–605.

Gunn, P. & Cuskelly, M. (1991). Down syndrome temperament: the stereotype at middle childhood and adolescence. *International Journal of Disability, Development and Education*, 38, 59–70.

Haeger, B. (1990). Mania in Down's syndrome (letter). *British Journal of Psychiatry*, 157, 153.

Hallidie-Smith, K.A. (1985). The heart. In *Current approaches to Down's syndrome*, ed. D. Lane & B. Stratford, pp. 52–70. London & New York: Holt, Rinehart & Winston.

Hannam, C. (1980). *Parents and mentally handicapped children*. Harmondsworth: Penguin.

Hanson, M.J. & Hanline, M.F. (1990). Parenting a child with a disability: a longitudinal study of parental stress and adaptation. *Journal of Early Intervention*, 14, 234–248.

Hart, D. & Walters, J. (1979). Brothers and sisters of mentally handicapped children. Unpublished report. Thomas Coram Research Unit, University of London.

Haslam, R.H.A. (1992). The physician and Down syndrome: are attitudes changing? *Journal of Child Neurology*, 7, 304–310.

*Heston, L.L. (1977). Alzheimer's disease, trisomy 21, and myeloproliferative disorders: associations suggesting a genetic diasthesis. *Science*, 196, 322–323.

Hewett, S. (1970). *The family and the handicapped child*. London: Allen & Unwin.

Hewitt, K.E., Carter G. & Jancar, J. (1985). Ageing in Down's syndrome. *British Journal of Psychiatry*, 147, 58–62.

Hindley, C.B. (1965). Stability and change in abilities up to five years. *Journal of Child Psychology and Psychiatry*, **6**, 85–99.

Hodes, R.J. (1994). Alzheimer's disease: treatment research finds new targets. *Journal of the American Geriatrics Society*, **42**, 679–681.

Holloway, S. & Brock, D.J.H. (1988). Changes in maternal age distribution and their possible impact on demand for prenatal diagnostic services. *British Medical Journal*, **296**, 978–981.

Holmes, N. (1988). The quality of life of mentally handicapped adults and their families. Unpublished Ph.D. thesis, University of London.

Holmes, N. & Carr, J. (1991). The pattern of care in families of adults with a mental handicap: a comparison between families of autistic adults and Down syndrome adults. *Journal of Autism and Developmental Disorders*, **12**, 159–176.

Holt, G.M., Bouras, N. & Watson, J.P. (1988). Down's syndrome and eating disorders. A case study. *British Journal of Psychiatry*, **152**, 847–848.

Holt, K.S. (1958). The home care of severely retarded children. *Pediatrics*, **22**, 744–755.

Hook, E.B. (1976). Estimates of maternal age specific risks of a Down-syndrome birth in women aged 34–41. *Lancet*, ii, 33–34.

*Hook, E.B. & Cross, P.K. (1982). Paternal age and Down's syndrome genotypes diagnosed prenatally: no association in New York State data. *Human Genetics*, **62**, 167–174.

Irwin, K.C. (1989). The school achievement of children with Down's syndrome. *New Zealand Medical Journal*, **102**, 11–13.

Jancar, J. (1988). Consequences of longer life for the mentally handicapped. *Geriatric Medicine*, May, 81–87.

Johnson, A.W. & Abelson, R.W. (1969). The behavioral competence of mongoloid and non-mongoloid retardates. *American Journal of Mental Deficiency*, **73**, 856–857.

Jones, D. & Casey, W. (1990). A longitudinal study of cognitive development and academic attainments in Down's syndrome children. *British Psychological Society Journal, Education Section*, **14**, 13–14.

Jones, D.C. & Lowry, R.B. (1975). Falling maternal age and incidence of Down syndrome (letter) *Lancet*, i, 753.

Kernan, K.T. (1990). Comprehension of syntactically indicated sequence by Down's syndrome and other mentally retarded adults. *Journal of Mental Deficiency Research*, **34**, 169–178.

Kirk, S.A. (1964). Research in education. In *Mental retardation: a review of research*, ed. H.A. Stevens & R. Heber, pp. 57–99. Chicago: University of Chicago Press.

Kirman, B. (1969). Mongols and their mothers. *Mental Retardation*, **1**, 57–74.

Kirman, B. (1975). Genetic errors: chromsome anomalies. In *Mental Handicap*, ed. B. Kirman & J. Bicknell, pp. 121–165. London: Churchill Livingstone.

Klederas, J.B., McIlvane, W.J. & McKay, H.A. (1989). Progressive decline of picture naming in an aging Down syndrome man with dementia. *Perceptual and Motor Skills*, **69**, 1091–1100.

Knight, L. (1988). Personal view. *British Medical Journal*, **296**, 567.

Knobloch, H. & Pasamanick, B. (1960). An evaluation of the consistency and predictive value of the 40-week Gesell developmental schedule. *Psychiatric Research Reports*, 13, 10–41.

Koch, R., Share, J. & Graliker, B.V. (1963). The predictability of Gesell developmental scales in mongolism. *Journal of Pediatrics*, 62, 93–97.

*Kostrzewski, J. (1965). The dynamics of intellectual and social development in Down's syndrome: results of experimental investigation. *Roczniki Filozoficzne*, 13, 5–32.

Kostrzewski, J. (1974). The dynamics of intellectual development in individuals with complete and incomplete trisomy of chromosome group G in the karyotype. *Polish Psychological Bulletin*, 5, 153–158.

*Lai, F. & Williams, R.S. (1989). A prospective study of Alzheimer's disease in Down syndrome. *Archives of Neurology*, 46, 849–853.

Landesman-Dwyer, S. (1981). Living in the community. *American Journal of Mental Deficiency*, 86, 223–234.

Lane, D. (1985). After school: work and employment for adults with Down's syndrome? In *Current approaches to Down's syndrome*, ed. D. Lane & B. Stratford, pp. 386–400. London & New York: Holt, Rinehart & Winston.

Lazarus, A., Jaffe, R.L. & Dubin, W.R. (1990). Electroconvulsive therapy and major depression in Down's syndrome. *Journal of Clinical Psychiatry*, 51, 422–425.

Leiter, R.G. (1980). *Leiter International Performance Scale; instruction manual.* Chicago: Stoelting & Co.

Lillie, T. (1993). A harder thing than triumph: roles of fathers of children with disabilities. *Mental Retardation*, 31, 438–443.

Lindsay, W.R., Michie, A.M., Baty, F.J. & Smith, A.H.W. (1988). A comprehensive programme for training social and community living skills: short term and long term results. Paper delivered at the 8th World Congress of the International Association for the Scientific Study of Mental Deficiency, Dublin, 21–25 August.

Lonsdale, G. (1978). Family life with a handicapped child: the parents speak. *Child: Care, Health and Development*, 4, 99–120.

Lorenz, S., Sloper, T. & Cunningham, C. (1985). Reading and Down's syndrome. *British Journal of Special Education*, 12, 65–67.

Ludlow, J.R. (1980). *Down's Syndrome – let's be positive.* Birmingham: Down's Children Association.

Ludlow, J.R. & Allen, L.M. (1979). The effect of early intervention and pre-school stimulus on the development of the Down's syndrome child. *Journal of Mental Deficiency Research*, 23, 29–44.

Lund, J. (1988). Psychiatric aspects of Down's syndrome. *Acta Psychiatrica Scandinavica*, 78, 369–374.

McConachie, H. & Domb, H. (1983). An interview study of 20 older brothers and sisters of mentally handicapped and non-handicapped children. *Mental Handicap*, 11, 64–66.

McGrother, C.W. & Marshall, B. (1990). Recent trends in incidence, morbidity and survival in Down's syndrome. *Journal of Mental Deficiency Research*, 34, 49–57.

Maksym, D. (1990). *Shared feelings*. Ontario: G. Allan, Roeher Institute, Kinsmen Building. (Obtainable through the Down's Syndrome Association.)

Marcell, M.M. & Weeks, S.L. (1988). Short-term memory difficulties and Down's syndrome. *Journal of Mental Deficiency Research*, 32, 153–62.

Meakin, C.J., Renvoize, E.B. & Kent, J. (1987). Folie à deux in Down's syndrome. A case report. *British Journal of Psychiatry*, 151, 258–260.

Melyn, M.A. & White, D.T. (1973). Mental and developmental milestones of non-institutionalised Down's syndrome children. *Pediatrics*, 52, 542–545.

Merrill-Palmer Scale of Mental Tests (1948). New York: Harcourt Brace & World.

Mittler, P.J. (1973). Purposes and principles of assessment. In *Assessment for learning in the mentally handicapped*, ed. P. Mittler, pp. 1–16. London: Churchill Livingstone.

Mittler, P.J. (1979). Patterns of partnership between parents and professionals. *Teaching and Training*, 17, 111–116.

Moore, B.C., Thuline, H.C. & Capes, L. (1968). Mongoloid and non-mongoloid retardates: a behavioral comparison. *American Journal of Mental Deficiency*, 73, 433–436.

Morgan, S.B. (1979). Adaptive skills in Down's syndrome children: implications for early intervention. *Mental Retardation*, 17, 247–249.

Murdoch, J.C. (1982). A survey of Down's syndrome under general practitioner care in Scotland. *Journal of the Royal College of General Practitioners*, 32, 410–418.

Murdoch, J.C. (1983). Communication of the diagnosis of Down's syndrome and spina bifida in Scotland, 1971–1981. *Journal of Mental Deficiency Research*, 27, 247–253.

Murdoch, J.C. (1985). Congenital heart disease as a significant factor in the morbidity of children with Down's syndrome. *Journal of Mental Deficiency Research*, 29, 147–151.

Murdoch, J.C. & Ogston, S.A. (1984). Down's syndrome children and parental upset. *Journal of the Royal College of General Practitioners*, 34, 87–90.

Myers, B.A. & Pueschel, S.M. (1991). Psychiatric disorders in persons with Down syndrome. *Journal of Nervous and Mental Disease*, 179, 609–613.

Neale, M.D. (1958). *Neale analysis of reading ability manual*. London: Macmillan.

Neumayer, R., Smith, R.W. & Lundegren, H.M. (1993). Leisure-related peer preference choices of individuals with Down's syndrome. *Mental Retardation*, 31, 396–402.

Newson, J. & Newson, E. (1963). *Infant care in an urban community*. London: Allen & Unwin.

Newson, J. & Newson, E. (1968). *Four years old in an urban community*. London: Allen & Unwin.

Newson, J. & Newson, E. (1976). *Seven years old in the home environment*. London: Allen & Unwin.

Newson, J. & Newson, E. (1977). *Perspectives on school at seven years*. London: Allen & Unwin.

Newson, J. & Newson, E. (1989). *The extent of parental physical punishment in the UK*. London: APPROACH (Association for the Protection of All Children).

Nicholson, A. & Alberman, E. (1992). Prediction of the number of Down's syndrome infants to be born in England and Wales up to the year 2000 and their likely survival rates. *Journal of Mental Deficiency Research*, **36**, 505–517.

Nilsson, I. (1988). Daily activities in the local community. Paper delivered at the 8th World Congress of the International Association for the Scientific Study of Mental Deficiency, Dublin, 21–5 August.

Nolan, M., McCartney, E., McArthur, K. & Rowson, V.R. (1980). A study of the hearing and receptive vocabulary of the trainees in an adult training centre. *Journal of Mental Deficiency Research*, **24**, 271–286.

O'Dwyer, J., Holmes, J. & Collacott, R.A. (1992). Two cases of obsessive-compulsive disorder in individuals with Down's syndrome. *Journal of Nervous and Mental Disease*, **180**, 603–604.

Oliver, C. & Holland, A.J. (1986). Down's syndrome and Alzheimer's disease: a review. *Psychological Medicine*, **16**, 307–322.

*Owens, J.R., Harris, F., Walker, S., McAllister, E. & West, L. (1983). The incidence of Down's syndrome over a 19 year period with special reference to maternal age. *Journal of Medical Genetics*, **20**, 90–93.

*Penrose, L.S. (1933). The relative effects of paternal and maternal age in mongolism. *Journal of Genetics*, **27**, 219–224.

Penrose, L.S. (1949). The incidence of mongolism in the general population. *Journal of Mental Science*, **95**, 685–688.

*Penrose, L.S. (1965). The causes of Down's syndrome. *Advances in Teratology*. London: Logos Press.

Penrose, L.S. & Smith, G.F. (1966). *Down's anomaly*. London: J. & A. Churchill.

*Pieterse, M. & Treloar, R. (1981). *The Down's syndrome program*. Progress Report, 1981, MacQuarie University.

Piper, M.C. & Pless, I.B. (1980). Early intervention for infants with Down syndrome: a controlled trial. *Pediatrics*, **65**, 463–468.

Pototzky, C. & Grigg, A.E. (1942). A revision of the prognosis in mongolism. *American Journal of Orthopsychiatry*, **12**, 503–510.

Prasher, V.P. (1994). Health in adults with Down syndrome. Thesis submitted to the Faculty of Medicine and Dentistry (Department of Psychiatry), University of Birmingham.

Prenderville, M. (1988). A friendship scheme for adults with mental handicap – an evaluation. Paper delivered at the 8th World Congress of the International Association for the Scientific Study of Mental Deficiency, Dublin, 21–25 August.

Pueschel, S.M. & Murphy, A. (1976). Assessment of counselling practices at the birth of a child with Down's syndrome. *American Journal of Mental Deficiency*, **81**, 325–330.

Putnam, J.W., Pueschel, S.M. & Holman, J.G. (1988). Community activities of youths and adults with Down's syndrome. *British Journal of Mental Subnormality*, **34**, 47–53.

Ramsay, M. & Piper, M.C. (1980). A comparison of two developmental scales in evaluating infants with Down syndrome. *Early Human Development*, **4**, 89–95.

Registrar General (1960). *Classification of Occupations*. London: HMSO.

Reynell, J. (1969). *Reynell Developmental Language Scale*. Slough, Bucks: National Foundation for Educational Research.

Richards, B.W. (1968). Is Down's syndrome a modern disease? *Lancet*, ii, 353–354.

Richardson, S.A., Koller, H. & Katz, M. (1985). Relationship of upbringing to later behavior disturbance of mildly mentally retarded young people. *American Journal of Mental Deficiency*, 90, 1–8.

*Richman, N., Stevenson, J. & Graham, P. (1982). *Pre-school to school – a behavioural study*. London: Academic Press.

Roberts, R.S., Sutton, E., Stroud, M., Ayidiya, S. & Davis, G. (1988). Use of quality of life scales to measure outcomes of a project using volunteers with elderly persons with mental retardation. Paper delivered at the 8th World Congress of the International Association for the Scientific Study of Mental Deficiency, Dublin, 21–25 August.

Rodgers, C. (1987). Maternal support for the Down's syndrome stereotype: the effect of direct experience of the condition. *Journal of Mental Deficiency Research* 31, 271–278.

Rodrigue, J.R., Morgan, S.B. & Geffken, G.R. (1992). Pychosocial adaptation of fathers of children with autism, Down syndrome, and normal development. *Journal of Autism and Developmental Disorders*, 22, 249–63.

Rollin, H.R. (1946). Personality in mongolism with special reference to the incidence of catatonic psychosis. *American Journal of Mental Deficiency*, 51, 219–237.

Ross, R.T. (1971). A preliminary study of self-help skills and age in hospitalized Down's syndrome patients. *American Journal of Mental Deficiency*, 76, 373–377.

*Rowe, R.D. & Uchida, I.A. (1961). Cardiac malformation in mongolism. *American Journal of Medicine*, 31, 726–735.

Rutter, M., Tizard, J. & Whitmore, K. (1970). *Education, health and behaviour*. London: Longman.

Ryde-Brandt, B. (1988). Mothers of primary school children with Down's syndrome: how do they experience their situation? *Acta Psychiatrica Scandinavica*, 78, 102–108.

Sawtell, M. (1993). *Healthy eating and exercise: information for older children and adults with Down's syndrome and their carers*. London: Down's Syndrome Association.

Saxby, H., Thomas, M., Felce, D. & de Kock, U. (1986). The use of shops, cafés, and public houses by severely and profoundly handicapped adults. *British Journal of Mental Subnormality*, 32, 215–220.

Schaie, K.W. (1983). What can we learn from the longitudinal study of adult psychological development? In *Longitudinal studies of adult psychological development*, ed. K.W. Schaie, pp 1–19. New York: Guilford Press.

Schnell, R.R. (1984). Psychomotor development. In *The young child with Down syndrome*, ed. S.M. Pueschel, pp. 207–226. New York: Human Sciences Press.

Seltzer, M.M., Krauss, M.W. & Tsunematsu, N. (1993). Adults with Down Syndrome and their aging mothers: diagnostic group differences. *American Journal on Mental Retardation*, **92**, 496–508.

Shah, A., Holmes, N. & Wing, L. (1982). Prevalence of autism and related conditions in adults in a mental handicap hospital. *Applied Research in Mental Retardation*, **8**, 303–317.

Shepperdson, B. (1984). Care of Down's syndrome teenagers. *Update*, 1 February, 370–372.

Shepperdson, B. (1992). A longitudinal study of Down's syndrome adults. End of Grant Award Report, Economic and Social Research Council, Swindon.

Shipe, D. & Shotwell, A.M. (1965). Effect of out-of-home care on mongoloid children: a continuation study. *American Journal of Mental Deficiency*, **69**, 649–652.

Shotwell, A.M. & Shipe, D. (1964). Effect of out-of-home care on the intellectual and social development of mongoloid children. *American Journal of Mental Deficiency*, **68**, 693–699.

Silverstein, A.B. (1964). An empirical test of the mongoloid stereotype. *American Journal of Mental Deficiency*, **68**, 493–497.

Silverstein, A.B., Ageno, D., Alleman, K.T., Derecho, K.T. & Gray, S.J. (1985). Adaptive behavior of institutionalized individuals with Down syndrome. *American Journal of Mental Deficiency*, **89**, 555–558.

Silverstein, A.B., Herbs, D., Miller, T.J., Nasuta, R. & Williams, D.L. (1988). Effects of age on the adaptive behavior of institutionalized and non-institutionalized individuals with Down's syndrome. *American Journal on Mental Retardation*, **92**, 455–460.

Silverstein, A.B., Herbs, D., Nasuta, R. & White, J.F. (1986). Effects of age on the adaptive behavior of institutionalized individuals with Down's syndrome. *American Journal of Mental Deficiency*, **90**, 659–662.

Sloper, P., Cunningham, C., Turner, S. & Knussen, C. (1990). Factors related to the academic attainments of children with Down's syndrome. *British Journal of Educational Psychology*, **60**, 284–298.

Sloper, P., Knussen, C., Turner, S. & Cunningham, C. (1991). Factors related to stress and satisfaction with life in families of children with Down's syndrome. *Journal of Child Psychology and Psychiatry*, **32**, 655–676.

Sovner, R., Hurley, A.D. & LaBrie, R. (1985). Is mania incompatible with Down's syndrome? *British Journal of Psychiatry*, **146**, 319–320.

Sports Council (1988). *Into the 90s: a strategy for sport for 1988–1993*. London: Sports Council.

Stallard, P. (1993). The behaviour of 3-year-old children: prevalence and parental perception of problem behaviour. *Journal of Child Psychology and Psychiatry*, **34**, 413–421.

Stedman, D.J. & Eichorn, D.H. (1964). A comparison of the growth and development of institutionalized and home-reared mongoloids during infancy and early childhood. *American Journal of Mental Deficiency*, **69**, 391–401.

Steele, J. (1993). Prenatal diagnosis and Down syndrome. Part 2. Possible effects. *Mental Handicap Research*, **6**, 57–69.

Stein, Z., Susser, M. & Gutterman, A.V. (1973). Screening programme for prevention of Down's syndrome. *Lancet*, i, 305–310.

*Stene, J., Stene, E., Stengel-Rutkowski, S. & Murken, J.D. (1981). Paternal age and Down's syndrome. Data from prenatal diagnosis (D.F.G.). *Human Genetics*, 59, 119–124.

Stratford, B. & Steele, J. (1985). Incidence and prevalence of Down's syndrome – a discussion and report. *Journal of Mental Deficiency Research*, 29, 95–107.

*Struwe, F. (1929). Histopathologische untersuchungen über enstehung und wesen der senilen plaques. *Zeitschrift für die gesamte Neurologie und Psychiatrie*, 122, 291–307.

Szymanski, L.S. & Biederman, J. (1984). Depression and anorexia nervosa of persons with Down syndrome. *American Journal of Mental Deficiency*, 89, 246–251.

Tew, B. & Laurence, K.M. (1975). Some sources of stress found in mothers of spina bifida children. *British Journal of Preventive and Social Medicine*, 29, 27–30.

Tew, B. & Laurence, K.M. (1983). The relationship between spina bifida children's intelligence test scores on school entry and at school leaving: a preliminary report. *Child: Care, Health and Development*, 9, 13–17.

Tew, B., Payne, H. & Laurence, K.M. (1974). Must a family with a handicapped child always be a handicapped family? *Developmental Medicine and Child Neurology*, 16, (Suppl. 32), 95–98.

Thase, M.E. (1982a) Reversible dementia in Down's syndrome. *Journal of Mental Deficiency Research*, 26, 111–113.

Thase, M.E. (1982b). Longevity and mortality in Down's syndrome. *Journal of Mental Deficiency Research*, 26, 177–192.

Thase, M.E. (1988). The relationship between Down syndrome and Alzheimer's disease. In *The psychobiology of Down syndrome*, ed. L. Nadel, pp. 345–368. Cambridge, MA: MIT Press.

Thomas, A. & Chess, S. (1977). *Temperament and development.* New York: Brunner-Mazel.

Thomas, A., Chess, S. & Birch, H.G. (1968). *Temperament and behaviour disorders in children.* London: University of London Press.

Tizard, J. & Grad, J.C. (1961). *The mentally handicapped and their families.* London: Oxford University Press.

Tredgold, A.F. (1937). *Text-book of mental deficiency,* 6th edition. London: Ballière, Tindall & Cox.

Tunali, B. & Power, T.G. (1993). Creating satisfaction: a psychological perspective on stress and coping in families of handicapped children. *Journal of Child Psychology and Psychiatry*, 34, 945–957.

Turnbull, A.P. & Turnbull, H.R. (1982). Parent involvement in the education of handicapped children: a critique. *Mental Retardation*, 20, 115–122.

Turner, R.K., Mathews, A. & Rachman, S. (1967). The stability of the WISC in a psychiatric group. *British Journal of Educational Psychology*, 37, 194–200.

Turner, S., Sloper, P., Cunningham, C. & Knussen, C. (1990). Health problems in children with Down's syndrome. *Child: Care, Health and Development*, 16, 83–97.

Turner, S., Sloper, P., Knussen, C. & Cunningham, C. (1991). Socio-economic factors: their relationship with child and family functioning for children with Down's syndrome. *Mental Handicap Research*, 4, 80–100.

Van Riper, M., Ryff, C. & Pridham, K. (1992). Parental and family well-being in families of children with Down's syndrome: a comparative study. *Research in Nursing and Health*, 15, 227–235.

Vernon, P. (1960). *Intelligence and attainment tests*. London: University of London Press.

Waisbren, S.E. (1980). Parents' reactions to the birth of a developmentally disabled child. *American Journal of Mental Deficiency*, 84, 345–351.

Wald, N.J. & Watt, H.C. (1994). Choice of serum markers in antenatal screening for Down's syndrome. *Journal of Medical Screening*, 1, 117–120.

*Walker, E.L. (1958). Action decrement and its relation to human learning. *Psychological Review*, 65, 129–142.

Wallin, J.E.W. (1944). Mongolism among school children. *American Journal of Orthopsychiatry*, 14, 104–112.

Ward, L. (1988). Developing community based services for people with mental handicaps. *Current Opinion in Psychiatry*, 1, 578–583.

Warren, A.C., Holroyd, S. & Folstein, M.F. (1989). Major depression in Down's syndrome. *British Journal of Psychiatry*, 155, 202–205.

Wechsler, D. (1967). *The Wechsler Pre-School and Primary Scale of Intelligence*. New York: Psychological Corporation.

Wing, L. (1980). MRC handicaps, behaviour and skills (HBS) schedule in epidemiological research. *Acta Psychiatrica Scandinavica*, Supplement 285, 62, 241–247.

Wing, L. & Gould, J. (1979). Severe impairments of social interaction and associated abnormalities in children: epidemiology and classification. *Journal of Autism and Developmental Disorders*, 9, 11–29.

Wishart, J. (1986). The effects of step-by-step training on cognitive performance in infants with Down's syndrome. *Journal of Mental Deficiency Research*, 30, 233–250.

Wishart, J. (1988). Early learning in infants and young children with Down's syndrome. In *The psychobiology of Down's syndrome*, ed L. Nadel, pp. 7–50. Boston, MA: M.I.T.P. Press.

Wishart, J. (1990). Learning to learn: the difficulties faced by infants and young children with Down's syndrome. In *Key issues in research in mental retardation*, ed. W.I. Fraser, pp. 249–269. London: Routledge.

Wishart, J.G. (1991). Early intervention. In *Halla's caring for people with mental handicap*, 8th edn, ed. W. Fraser, R. MacGillvray & A. Green, pp. 21–27. London: Butterworth.

Wishart, J. & Johnston, F.H. (1990). The effects of experience on attribution of a stereotyped personality to children with Down's syndrome. *Journal of Mental Deficiency Research*, 34, 409–420.

*Wisniewski, K.E., Wisniewski, H.M. & Wen, G.Y. (1985). Occurrence of neuropathological changes and dementia of Alzheimer's disease in Down's syndrome. *Annals of Neurology*, 17, 278–282.

*Witty, P.A. & McCafferty, E. (1930). Attainment by feebleminded children. *Education*, 50, 588–597.

Wolff, L.C., Noh, S., Fisman, S.N. & Speechley, M. (1989). Brief report: psychological effects of parenting stress on parents of autistic children. *Journal of Autism and Developmental Disorders*, **19**, 157–166.

Yamamoto, K., Soliman, A., Parsons, J. & Davies, O.L. Jr (1987). Voices in unison: stressful events in the lives of children in six countries. *Journal of Child Psychology and Psychiatry*, **28**, 855–864.

Yeates, S. (1992). Have they got a hearing loss? *Mental Handicap*, **20**, 126–133.

Yule, W., Gold, R.D. & Busch, C. (1982). Long-term predictive validity of the WPPSI: an 11-year follow-up study. *Personality and Individual Differences*, **3**, 65–71.

Zaremba, J. (1985). Recent medical research. In *Current approaches to Down's syndrome*, ed. D. Lane & B. Stratford, pp. 27–54. London & New York: Holt, Rinehart & Winston.

Zellweger, H. (1968). Is Down's syndrome a modern disease? *Lancet*, **ii**, 458.

Zigman, W.B., Schupf, N., Silverman, W.P. & Sterling, R.C. (1989). Changes in adaptive functioning of adults with developmental disabilities. *Australian and New Zealand Journal of Developmental Disabilities*, **15**, 277–287.

Index